Benzodiazepines

Benzodiazepines

Edited by

MICHAEL R. TRIMBLE

*Professor of Behavioural Neurology, Institute of Neurology, and
Consultant Physician in Psychological Medicine,
National Hospitals for Neurology and Neurosurgery, London, UK*

and

IAN HINDMARCH

*Professor of Human Psychopharmacology and Head of the HPRU,
Medical Research Centre, University of Surrey, Guildford, UK*

WRIGHTSON BIOMEDICAL PUBLISHING LTD

Petersfield, UK and Philadelphia, USA

Copyright © 2000 by Wrightson Biomedical Publishing Ltd

Editorial Office:

Wrightson Biomedical Publishing Ltd
Ash Barn House, Winchester Road, Stroud,
Petersfield, Hampshire GU32 3PN, UK
Telephone: 44 (0)1730 265647
Fax: 44 (0)1730 260368

British Library Cataloguing in Publication Data
Benzodiazepines
   1. Benzodiazepines 2. Benzodiazepines – Therapeutic use –
   Effectiveness 3. Benzodiazepines – Therapeutic use – Side
   effects
   I. Trimble, Michael R. II. Hindmarch, I. (Ian)
   615.7'882

Library of Congress Cataloging in Publication Data
A catalog record for this book is available from the Library of Congress

ISBN 1 871816 43 2

Composition by Scribe Design, Gillingham, Kent
Printed in Great Britain by Biddles Ltd, Guildford

Contents

Contributors

Christer Allgulander, *Neurotec, Section of Psychiatry, M57 Huddinge University Hospital, S-141 86 Huddinge, Sweden*

Kailash P. Bhatia, *Department of Clinical Neurology, Institute of Neurology, Queen Square, London WC1N 3BG, UK*

George Beaumont, *Visiting Professor, HPRU, University of Surrey, Guildford, UK*

H. Valerie Curran, *Clinical Health Psychology, University College London, Gower Street, London WC1E 6BT, UK*

Morgan Feely, *Department of Medicine, Martin Wing, Leeds General Infirmary, Leeds LS1 3EX, UK*

Alan Guberman, *Division of Neurology, University of Ottawa, The Ottawa Hospital, General Campus, 501 Smyth Road, Ottawa, Ontario, Canada K1H 8L6*

James Lavett, *Raymond Way Neuropsychiatry Unit, Queen Square, London WC1N 3BG, UK*

Brian E. Leonard, *Pharmacology Department, National University of Ireland, Galway, Ireland*

John H. Livingston, *Department of Paediatric Neurology, Leeds General Infirmary, Leeds LS2 9NS, UK*

Anthony N. Nicholson, *Centre for Human Sciences, Defence Evaluation and Research Agency, Farnborough, Hampshire, GU14 6SZ, UK*

J.W. Sander, *University Department of Clinical Neurology, Institute of Neurology, Queen Square, London WC1N 3BG, UK*

Caroline E. Selai, *Raymond Way Neuropsychiatry Unit, Institute of Neurology, Queen Square, London WC1N 3BG, UK*

J. Smith, *Department of Psychiatry, Cefn Coed Hospital, Swansea SA2 0GH, UK*

Michael R. Trimble, *Raymond Way Neuropsychiatry Unit, Institute of Neurology, Queen Square, London WC1N 3BG, UK*

M.C. Walker, *University Department of Clinical Neurology, Institute of Neurology, Queen Square, London WC1N 3BG, UK*

D.D.R. Williams, *Department of Psychiatry, Cefn Coed Hospital, Swansea SA2 0GH, UK*

Preface

Benzodiazepines, since their serendipitous discovery in the late 1950s, have proved to be one of the most useful groups of medicinal agent within psychopharmacology where psychiatric disorders and neurological conditions need pharmacological management. Patients with anxiety, sleep disturbance, panic, alcoholism, those needing premedication for surgery and unpleasant dental procedures, and those needing muscle relaxation are among the nurmerous and major beneficiaries of medicines from the benzodiazepine group of drugs.

Benzodiazepines augment the activity of GABA, one of the most widespread inhibiting neurotransmitters, and this arguably gives them their unrivalled spectrum of clinical activity, as well as producing the unwanted side-effects of sedation, amnesia and impaired psychomotor function with which some of the molecules are associated.

There exist, however, benzodiazepine derivatives and benzodiazepine-like ligands of the GABA-Cl ion receptor complex which, by their intrinsic pharmacological nature are anticonvulsant and anxiolytic without being sedative or amnesic (e.g. clobazam), hypnotic-sedatives without next morning residual effects (e.g. triazolam, temazepam, loprazolam and zopiclone), non-sedative hypnotics (e.g. zaleplon), hypnotics without anti-anxiety effects (e.g. zopiclone), and at the same time, anti-anxiety agents with sedative, amnesic, anticonvulsant, and myorelaxant activity (e.g. lorazepam, diazepam). The differences between the various molecules are no doubt accounted for by the specific binding characteristics of each drug and by their profile on a continuum encompassing full agonists, through antagonists to inverse agonists.

While the early chapters of the book examine the pharmacological properties of benzodiazepines, their amnesic activity and their utility in the management of anxiety and sleep disturbance, later chapters relate to the use of benzodiazepines in epilepsy. It was considerably unfortunate, amidst the political turmoil and confusion about the use of benzodiazepines in psychiatry, that their very valuable use in the management of patients with neurological conditions was overlooked. This had the consequences of denying the use of benzodiazepines to many patients who may have benefited from them, adding the fearful prospect of patients who did not use them for epilepsy being told that they were likely to be regarded as drug addicts. This has been singularly unhelpful. Further, the withdrawal of investment in the benzodiazepines by the pharmaceutical industry has led to a failure to follow up the potentially exciting lines for the development of new anticpileptic drugs, particularly the partial agonists. Nonetheless, in spite of the considerable difficulties that benzodiazepines ran into some 10 years ago, they have continued to remain an important cornerstone in the management of epilepsy, and this is discussed here by several experts in the field. Perhaps of most importance has been the distinction between the rather more sedative 1,4-benzodiazepines, and the less sedative 1,5-benzodiazepines. The latter appear to have significant benefits for the management of epilepsy, which include not only the long half-life, but also probably active metabolic products, which help sustain the anticonvulsant activity.

It is hoped that reviewing this literature on the use of benzodiazepines in epilepsy will lead readers once again to appreciate the importance of these compounds in this management setting. During a recent workshop, the authors of the chapters in the epilepsy section of this book reached the collowing consensus.

1. Benzodiazepines have a clear role in the management of epilepsy. They are very beneficial in the treatment of status epilepticus and have a long-standing and well-established role in the oral management of epilepsy.
2. There are distinctions to be drawn between the 1,4- and 1,5-benzodi-azepines.
3. If a patient has been on a 1,4-benzodiazepine, and it has not been effec-tive, another benzodiazepine may be used. This involves switching to a 1,5-benzodiazepine. The converse is also true: patints who have failed on a 1,5-benzodiazepine may respond to a 1,4-benzodiazepine.
4. Benzodiazepines, particularly clobazam, can be effective in the manage-ment of non-convulsive status epilepticus.
5. With regard to convulsive status epilepticus, benzodiazepines are of value in all phases. Early on, rectal benzodiazepines are useful, if possible, diazepam. Buccal midazolam is a useful alternative. The use of benzodi-azepines such as intravenous lorazepam for established convulsive status is rcommended, and for later stages, midazolam infusions may be an alter-native treatment.
6. There is a role for the use of 1,5-benzodiazepines in the management of postictal behaviour disorders, in particular postictal psychoses.
7. Benzodiazepines, particularly 1,5-benzodiazepines, have been shown to be useful for intermittent short-term seizure therapy. This includes clusters of seizures to prevent the cluster developing and catamenial seizures. Further, benzodiazepines are useful in social situations, e.g. a wedding, where patients require short-term confidence that they are not going to have a seizure. They can be used in febrile episodes in children, and where patients have serial attacks of seizures heralding a possible status epilepticus.
8. The myclonic and startle symptoms of epilepsy respond to clonazepam.

With regard to the use of the 1,5-benzodiazepine, clobazam, further consensus was reached, as follows. This drug should be considered as first add-on therapy for patients with partial epilepsy when patients have failed to respond to standard therapies. Secondly, it has established value for the management of intermittent short-term seizure clusters, non-convulsive status epilepticus, and in patients where there is a subtle, and difficult to dissect, combination of epilepsy and anxiety states.

The issue of tolerance to benzodiazepines in general, but to clobazam in particular, is discussed at length. The consensus figure for the development of tolerance to the anticonvulsant effects of clobazam is between 30 and 50%. The consensus for those patients who develop sustained periods of seizure freedom in partial epilepsy with clobazam was 10–15%.

In this book, we have also included a chapter on the use of benzodiazepines in movement disorders. This essentially, is to remind readers that benzodiazepines are used in neurology beyond epilepsy. Indeed, with the ubiquitous distribution of the benzodiazepine receptor in the central nervous system, and a spectrum of activity which can range from inverse agonism to full agonism, the potential for the use of benzodiazepines in neurological practice is wider than is generally subsumed, even by neurologists.

The final chapter of the book provides a rational look at one of the aspects of the use of benzodiazepines – their potential to produce addiction – most frequently featured in media and non-scientific, lay journals. It is indeed sad that patients with morbid anxiety, sleep disturbance, neurological disorder, etc., should be stigmatized as 'drug addicts' when legitimately prescribed a benzodiazepine medication, and it is hoped that this volume will remind physicians that the benzodiazepines remain some of the most useful therapeutic agents for a wide variety of distressing and disabling psychiatric, general medical and neurological conditions.

The Editors and grateful to all the contributors to the book for their efforts in providing manuscripts, and particularly hope that, with the turn of the Millennium, benzodiazepines will contine to be seen as highly effective therapeutic agents, that their use will not simply be restricted to anxiety disorders, and that they will be acknowledged as truly neuropsychotropic agents which require further investment and exploration.

M. TRIMBLE, I. HINDMARCH
London and Guildford, July, 2000

Benzodiazepines
Edited by Michael R. Trimble and Ian Hindmarch
© 2000 Wrightson Biomedical Publishing Ltd

1

A Review of the Pharmacological Properties of the Benzodiazepine Anxiolytics

BRIAN E. LEONARD

Pharmacological Department, National University of Ireland, Galway, Ireland

The history of psychopharmacology is littered with examples of the impact of serendipity and drug development and nowhere is this more apparent than in the development of the benzodiazepines. These drugs, exemplified by chlordiazepoxide and diazepam, were shown to have anxiolytic properties in conventional animal models of anxiety and were subsequently marketed for some 20 years before they were discovered to produce their effects by modulating the action of the inhibitory transmitter gamma-aminobutyric acid (GABA) on the GABA-A receptors (see Sternbach, 1983). Following the discovery by Squires and Braestrup, and by Mohler and Okada, in 1997, that the benzodiazepines activated a specific modulatory site on the GABA-A receptor, numerous ligands have been developed that either increase or decrease the activity of GABA on the GABA-A receptor. Strictly speaking, the sites that the benzodiazepines act upon are not receptor sites but GABA modulatory sites. Furthermore, many non-benzodiazepines (such as the cyclopyrrolones, the pyrazolines, the beta-carbolines and the triazolopyridines) act on the benzodiazepine modulatory site. Thus, the term 'benzodiazepine receptor', while conventionally used, is incorrect because it is not a receptor in the conventional sense and non-benzodiazepine ligands act on it. However, for ease of communication the term 'benzodiazepine receptor' will be used in this chapter.

The purpose of this chapter is to discuss the relationship between the pharmacological properties of the benzodiazepines in terms of their actions on the benzodiazepine receptor and in particular to pay attention to the possible clinical advantages of partial benzodiazepine-receptor agonists in combining the beneficial anxiolytic effects with a lower tendency to cause cognitively impairing side effects.

GABA, BENZODIAZEPINES AND THE NEURO-ANATOMICAL BASIS OF ANXIETY

Polc and colleagues (1974) showed that the GABA agonist amino-oxyacetic acid, which acts by inhibiting the metabolism of GABA and raises the brain concentration of the amino acid five-fold, not only mimicked the action of diazepam on the spinal cord, but also enhanced the action of the benzodiazepine. These effects could be blocked by the GABA antagonist bicuculline and the GABA-synthesis inhibitor thiosemicarbazide. However, it was soon shown that these changes in GABA synthesis were not reflected in the anti-anxiety effects of the GABA agonist. Thus, Cook and Stepinwall (1975) showed that amino-oxyacetic acid did not shown any anxiolytic effects in rats that were subject to punished behaviour in a modified Geller–Seifter test. Furthermore, no syner-getic effects were found between diazepam and the GABA agonist. Similar findings were reported with the GABA agonist muscimol, while clinical trials with the GABA mimetic anticonvulsant progabide produced only weak anxiolytic effects. Such findings support the hypothesis that the benzodiazepines enhance the affinity of GABA for its receptors, particularly when the activity of the GABAergic system is suboptimal, but that raising the GABA concentration in the brain alone does not ensure that the transmitter is functionally active.

GABA-A receptors are widely distributed throughout the mammalian brain where they not only form part of the central inhibitory system but also modulate the catecholaminergic, serotonergic and cholinergic systems. The physiological actions of GABA are therefore very complex, so the enhance-ment of its activities by the benzodiazepines is likely to be a composite of the changes that occur in a large number of interconnected neurotransmitter processes. Nevertheless, there is evidence to suggest that the benzodiazepines that modulate GABA-A receptors in the cerebellum mediate the ataxic effects of the drugs, while those in the hypothalamus reduce the release of corticotrophin (ACTH) and enhance that of growth hormone. The forebrain and hippocampus are responsible for the amnesic properties while the amygdala, hippocampus and other limbic areas mediate the anticonflict and anxiolytic effects. The sedative properties of the benzodiazepines appear to reside in the reticular formation. The evidence for the anatomical sites of action of the benzodiazepines is largely based on experimental studies but, with the advent of imaging techniques in man, it should be possible to show whether similar regional changes also occur in the human brain.

HOW DO BENZODIAZEPINE-RECEPTOR LIGANDS AUGMENT GABA FUNCTION?

Electrophysiological studies showed that diazepam could potentiate the inhibitory effects of GABA. Later it was shown that the effect of diazepam could be abolished if the endogenous GABA content was depleted, thus establishing that diazepam, and related benzodiazepines, did not act directly on GABA receptors but in some way modulated inhibitory transmission via GABA (Polc and Haefely, 1977). Two groups of investigators were responsible for explaining how the benzodiazepines modulate GABAergic transmission at the molecular level (Costa *et al.*, 1975; Haefely *et al.*, 1975). These investigators showed that the benzodiazepines bind with high affinity and specificity to neuronal elements in the mammalian brain and that there was an excellent correlation between the affinity of the benzodiazepines for their specific binding sites and their pharmacological potencies in alleviating anxiety in both man and animals (Braestrup and Squires, 1978). The binding of a benzodiazepine to this receptor site is enhanced in the presence of GABA or a GABA agonist, thereby suggesting that a functional, but independent, relationship exists between the GABA receptor and the benzodiazepine receptor.

It is now established that GABA-A receptors comprise five classes of subunits (alpha, beta, gamma, delta and pi), which can be divided into at least 16 different subunit receptors (e.g. α-1 to α-6 in the mammalian brain (Mohler *et al.*, 1990; Leonard, 1993). There is evidence that three of these subunits (alpha, beta and gamma) are required for the responsiveness of the receptor to GABA or the 'classical' full agonist benzodiazepines.

Two distinct classes of receptors for GABA exist in the mammalian brain: GABA-A and GABA-B receptors. These are characterized by their affinity for specific agonist and antagonists, the effect or system to which they are coupled and the presence or absence of allosteric modulatory sites. Whereas the GABA-A receptors are linked to ion channels that regulate the chloride conductance of the subsynaptic membrane, GABA-B receptors are coupled to GTP binding proteins that regulate adenylate cyclase in addition to potassium and calcium channels (Bowery, 1989). GABA is the natural agonist for both types of receptors but selective agonists and antagonists exist which enable these receptor types to be distinguished. Thus, muscimol and baclofen are agonists, while bicuculline and phaclofen are antagonists of the GABA-A and GABA-B receptors respectively (Bowery, 1993; Johnson, 1991).

Allosteric sites on neuronal GABA-A receptors are targets through which benzodiazepines and benzodiazepine ligands such as the cyclopyrrolone zopiclone and the imidazopyridine zolpidem modulate GABA-A-receptor function. Other allosteric sites on the GABA-A receptor include those for the barbiturates, convulsants (such as picrotoxin) and general anaesthetics as exemplified by halothane, propofol, some steroids and ethanol (Ticku, 1991). A unique feature of the GABA-A receptor is its ability to mediate opposite pharmacological effects by facilitating or impeding GABA-receptor function, depending on the nature of the receptor ligand that binds to the allosteric sites. These modulatory effects are limited in their intensity, such that the

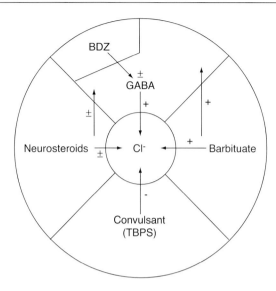

Figure 1. Binding sites on the GABA-A–benzodiazepine-receptor complex. (After Malizia and Nutt, 1995.)

maximal response to the physiological effects of GABA is not exceeded. This property of the GABA-A receptor is probably one of the primary reasons why agonists of the benzodiazepine receptor have a high therapeutic index.

Figure 1 is a diagrammatic representation of the different allosteric sites that have been identified on the GABA-A receptor.

The barbiturates, and to some extent alcohol, also seem to produce their anxiolytic and sedative effect by facilitating GABAergic transmission. This action of chemically unrelated compounds (i.e. alcohol, barbiturates and benzo-diazepines) can be explained by their abilities to stimulate specific sites on the GABA-receptor complex, the most marked effect being due to the benzo-diazepines when they activate their specific receptor site (Olsen and Venter, 1980; Tallman and Gallagher, 1985). Thus, benzodiazepines bind with high affinity to the benzodiazepine receptor and, as a result, change the structural conformation of the GABA receptor so that the action of GABA on its recep-tor is enhanced. This enables GABA to produce a stronger inhibition of the post-synaptic neuron than would occur in the absence of the benzodiazepine. The relationship between the various components of the GABA receptor and the actions of various benzodiazepine ligands on the GABA–benzodiazepine receptor complex has been discussed in detail by Haefely (1990).

The inhibitory effect of GABA is mediated by chloride ion channels. When the GABA receptor is occupied by GABA, or a drug acting as an agonist such as muscimol, the ion channels open and chloride ions together with potassium ions diffuse into the cell. Thus, an inhibitory transmitter like GABA thereby hyperpolarizes the cell. The chloride ion channel contains at least two binding sites. One of these sites is activated by barbiturates that have weak anxiolytic and hypnotic properties (e.g. pentobarbitone and phenobarbitone). Such drugs facilitate inhibitory transmission by increasing the duration of opening of the chloride ion channel. Another class of experimental anxiolytic agents that are not structurally related to the benzodiazepines, the pyrazolopyridines, of which etazolate is a clinically active example, also act as a specific site within the chloride ion channel and enhance GABAergic function by increasing the frequency of channel opening (Collins et al., 1976).

Thus, it may be concluded that the 'classical' benzodiazepines, such as diazepam, act as anxiolytics by activating a specific benzodiazepine receptor which facilitates inhibitory GABAergic transmission. Other drugs with anxiolytic properties, such as some of barbiturates and alcohol, also facilitate GABAergic transmission by acting on sites associated directly within the chloride ion channel.

THE CLINICAL IMPORTANCE OF BENZODIAZEPINE PARTIAL AGONISTS

While full agonists of the benzodiazepine receptor (such as diazepam and the other 1,4-benzodiazepines) produce their full range of pharmacological effects (namely anxiolysis, sedation, anticonvulsant effects and muscle relaxation) by occupying less than 50% of the benzodiazepine receptors, partial agonists cannot produce the full range of pharmacological effects even when 100% of the benzodiazepine receptors are occupied (see Potier et al., 1988). For example, the partial agonist bretazenil does not produce more than 25% of the potentiation action of GABA even though all the benzodiazepine receptors are fully occupied (Facklam et al., 1992). Thus, the partial agonists may provide a valuable addition to the clinically available benzodiazepines in that they appear to combine the useful properties of the conventional benzodiazepines (anxiolysis) without causing undue sedation, muscle relaxation or amnesia.

Apart from the partial agonists that are in the process of development, the 1,5-benzodiazepine clobazam is unique in that its relative lack of side effects (sedation, impaired psychomotor function etc.) has been associated with its partial agonist properties. These differences between clobazam and the conventional benzodiazepines may be attributed to the consequences of moving the diazepine ring nitrogen from the fourth to the fifth position. Thus, it has been shown that saturation of the imine double bond (i.e. C=N group in the diazepine ring) of the 1,4-benzodiazepines results in a loss of the anticonvulsant and muscle relaxant properties (Sternbach *et al.*, 1986). In contrast, the pharmacological activity of clobazam is not dependent on the presence of an imine group in the diazepine ring. This subtle change in the structure of the benzodiazepine molecule may confer the unique pharmacological properties on clobazam and help to place it in the partial agonist rather than the full agonist category. The main metabolite of clobazam in man, dog and monkey is *N*-desmethylclobazam (Volz *et al.*, 1979). Although it would appear that the clobazam metabolite is an active antiepileptic, it is less potent than the parent compound as an anxiolytic and has weaker sedative properties (Fielding and Hoffman, 1979). However, once the steady state concentration has been attained, the plasma concentration of the *N*-desmethyl metabolite is approximately eight times greater than that of the parent compound; the metabolite also has a much longer half-life than the parent drug (Koeppen, 1985).

This may account for the improved therapeutic profile of clobazam over the conventional 1,4-benzodiazepines as shown by its inability to impair saccadic eye movement velocity and other psychomotor and cognitive measures in man (vander Meyen *et al.*, 1989; Hindmarch 1995). Furthermore, electroencephalogram (EEG) and receptor affinity studies suggest that clobazam (and its desmethyl metabolite) may be partial agonists of benzodiazepine receptors at least in the rat brain (Mandenna *et al.*, 1991). There is experimental evidence to show that *N*-desmethylclobazam is a partial agonist (Noggin and Callaghan, 1985).

From these clinical and experimental studies it may be concluded that clobazam owes its improved therapeutic effect over the conventional benzodiazepines to its partial agonist action, a property that may be conferred by moving the nitrogen in the diazepine ring from the fourth to the fifth position. A detailed description of the clinical pharmacology of clobazam is given by Hindmarch (1995), Robertson (1995) and Beaumont (1995).

DIVERSITY OF DRUGS ACTING ON THE BENZODIAZEPINE RECEPTOR

Until about 1980, it was widely accepted that the benzodiazepine structure was a prerequisite for the anxiolytic profile and the recognition and binding to the benzodiazepine receptor. More recently, however, a chemically unrelated drug, the cyclopyrrolone zopiclone, which has a benzodiazepine-like profile, has been shown to be a useful sedative–hypnotic. Other chemical classes of drugs that are also structurally dissimilar to the benzodiazepines (e.g. the triazolopyridazines) have also been developed and shown to have anxiolytic activity in man; these non-benzodiazepines also act via the benzodiazepine receptor (Haefely *et al.*, 1985). Thus, the term 'benzodiazepine-

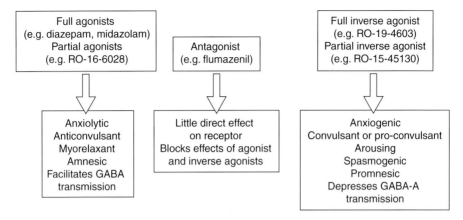

Figure 2. Properties of benzodiazepine-receptor ligands.

receptor ligand' has been introduced to describe all drugs, irrespective of their chemical structure, that act on benzodiazepine receptors and thereby modulate inhibitory transmission in the brain. The pharmacological properties of these different types of benzodiazepine receptor ligands are summarized in Figure 2.

At the molecular level, the differences between the agonist and antagonist benzodiazepines are ascribed to the ability of the drug to induce a conformational change in the fine structure of the receptor molecule that produces functional consequences in terms of the cellular changes. The partial agonists have intrinsic activity that lies between the full agonists and the antagonists. When administered they have qualitatively similar effects to full agonists but may not be quite as potent. When given with full agonists they reduce the potency of the full agonist. Some 16 years ago, the Danish investigators Braestrup and Nielsen (1983) found that a group of non-benzodiazepine compounds, the beta-carbolines, not only antagonized the actions of the full agonists but also had intrinsic activity themselves. Such compounds were clearly not pure antagonists, which lack intrinsic activity, but were found to be inverse agonists because they had the exact opposite biological effects to the pure agonists, i.e. they caused anxiety, convulsions and were promnesic.

Regions of the mammalian brain that are innervated by GABAergic neurons contain a high density of GABA-A receptors and its associated binding sites. The application of quantitative receptor autoradiographic methods has led to the identification of selective binding sites. These include high and low affinity sites for GABA, as well as the sites for benzodiazepine ligands and the modulatory sites associated directly with the chloride ion channel. The identification of these different sites has led to the conclusion that there are at least four main subtypes of the GABA-A receptor (Richards *et al.*, 1991). Encoded by a family of at least 15 genes, GABA-A-receptor subtypes are assembled from several subunits termed α-1 and α-6, β-1, β-4 and γ-1, γ-3, δ and π. Immunoprecipitation studies with subunit specific antibodies have shown that the most prevalent subunits (α-1, β-2, β-3 and γ-2) are frequently co-assembled to form a basic structure for most of the GABA-A receptors (Benke *et al.*, 1991). It is now known that different populations of neurons may be distinguished by specific GABA-A-receptor subtypes. For example, the α-1 subunit is frequently localized in GABAergic neurons, whereas monoaminergic and cholinergic neurons, which are modulated by GABAergic neurons, selectively express the α-3 subunit (Mohler and Fritschy, 1992). Based on the differences in the basic structure of the GABA-A receptors, four classes of receptor have been identified owing to their interactions with different types of benzodiazepine-receptor ligands. Type 1 receptors, with the structure of α-1, β, γ-2, show a high affinity for the imidazopyridine zolpidem. Type 2 receptors, with the subunit structure α-1, β, γ-2, have an intermediate affinity for zolpidem, while Type 3 receptors (α-5, β, γ-2) have a very low affinity for zolpidem. By contrast, Type 4 receptors (α-6, β, γ-2) have a low affinity for 1,4-benzodiazepine receptor agonists, but a high affinity for the inverse agonist RO 15-4513. It would appear that the type of γ subunit strongly influences the affinities of the receptor for antagonists and inverse agonists (Richards *et al.*, 1991).

At the subcellular level, it has been postulated that the GABA receptor might spontaneously oscillate between states of high and low affinity for GABA. It would appear that agonists and inverse agonists stabilize the receptor in the high and low affinity conformation respectively. Conversely, competitive antagonists might be unable to distinguish between these two conformational states but act by preventing the access of either the positive or negative allosteric modulators. Partial agonists, by contrast, produce a shift in the equilibrium between the low and high affinity state that is less marked than the full agonist because they cannot so readily distinguish between the two conformations.

The interaction between benzodiazepine-receptor ligands and their allosteric sites on the GABA-A-receptor complex is determined by its binding affinity and its intrinsic efficacy. Full agonists have positive intrinsic efficacy, inverse agonists have negative intrinsic efficacy, while between these extremes competitive antagonists have zero efficacy. The intrinsic efficacy of a benzodiazepine-receptor ligand may be quantified by measuring the GABA-stimulated chloride flux; such changes are directly reflected in the pharmacological profile of the ligand. For example, the 1,4- benzodiazepines such as diazepam are anxiolytic, sedative, muscle relaxants and anticonvulsants, whereas the full inverse agonists such as the beta-carboline DMCM have opposite effects.

The benzodiazepine receptor is unique in that it has a bi-directional function. This discovery could be of major importance in designing drugs in which the adverse effects of the 'classical' benzodiazepines could be reduced but their beneficial effects maintained. Although the 1,4-benzodiazepine anxiolytics are effective and safe drugs with a rapid onset of action, there is a practical need for drugs that are less sedative, with a lower dependence potential and a lack of interaction with alcohol. Similarly, the benzodiazepine hypnotics are liable to cause hangover effects, show a liability to tolerance development following prolonged use, cause amnesia and have an abuse potential (Lopez et al., 1990). It is possible that partial agonists may offer therapeutic advantages over the conventional full agonists; like clobazam, the partial agonist bretazenil has pharmacological properties that appear to support this hypothesis. Thus, it has been shown to produce only a mild degree of sedation at doses that are far higher than those which are anticonvulsant and which have marked anticonflict effects. Bretazenil shows little interaction with ethanol but antagonizes the sedative and motor impairing effects of high doses of diazepam. In animal studies, there is little evidence of physical dependence (Haefely et al., 1990). Preliminary clinical studies also suggest that bretazenil is an effective anxiolytic with a lower propensity to cause sedation, muscle relaxation and amnesia than diazepam. The abuse potential also appears to be low (Delini-Stula, 1992). While these preliminary clinical studies suggest that bretazenil is not entirely devoid of undesirable properties, it does show a higher therapeutic index than the 'classical' benzodiazepines. Thus, the development of partial agonists may be particularly important in the production of anxiolytics that lack the sedative and amnesic properties of agonists.

NOVEL BENZODIAZEPINE RECEPTOR LIGANDS WITH POSSIBLE SELECTIVE ANXIOLYTIC PROPERTIES

Following the discovery of receptor sites for the benzodiazepines in the mammalian brain, a wide variety of chemical structures has been identified that also interact with these allosteric sites on the GABA-A receptor. These include the beta-carbolines, the triazolopyridines, the pyrrazolines and the imidazopyridines. The first of these novel compounds to be described was the cyclopyrrolone zopiclone. Later, analogues of zopiclone were developed (such as suriclone and sulproclone), which were found to have a higher affinity for the benzodiazepine-receptor site.

The effect of drugs on the GABA-evoked chloride channel opening may be quantified by measuring their effect on the binding of 35S-TBPS to rat brain membranes. TBPS is a chemical probe that binds to a site in the interior of the open chloride channel of the GABA-A receptor, the degree of binding of TBPS thereby giving a measure of the extent of channel opening. In this model, drugs such as diazepam, zopiclone, zolpidem and suriclone enhance 35S-TBPS binding while inverse agonists, such as DMCM, decrease it. These results suggest that the cyclopyrrolones are full agonists on the benzodiazepine–GABA receptor complex. Further studies showed that these drugs did not discriminate between the benzodiazepine type 1 (Bz1) and type 2 (Bz2) receptor sites. However, some investigators have provided experimental evidence to show that the cyclopyrrolones and the benzodiazepines bind to two distinct but allosterically coupled sites on the GABA-A receptor (Trifiletti and Snyder, 1984). These investigators further suggested that the binding of the cyclopyrrolones led to the formation of a different conformational state of the GABA receptor from that occurring after the binding of the benzodiazepines. Other experimental studies have shown that the temperature sensitivity of bindings of the cyclopyrrolones is different from the 'classical' benzodiazepines such as diazepam but similar to the triazolobenzodiazepines that also have sedative and anxiolytic properties (Chweh et al., 1985).

To what extent are the biochemical differences between the cyclopyrrolones such as zopiclone and suriclone and the 'classical' benzodiazepines reflected in their pharmacological differences? There is experimental evidence to show that zopiclone induces slow wave sleep and increases the duration of slow wave sleep in rats, but that unlike nitrazepam or the triazolobenzodiazepine triazolam, it does not depress rapid eye movement (REM) sleep (Julou et al., 1983). In healthy volunteers, zopiclone has also been shown to have a similar effect (Musch and Maillard, 1990). Furthermore, the relatively short duration of action (6–7 h) with a relatively little adverse effect on sleep architecture may explain the low residual effect of the drug on waking. Compared with the long half-life benzodiazepines such as nitrazepam, zopiclone does not significantly affect daytime vigilance, psychomotor performance or produce amnesia the day after taking the drug (Musch and Maillard, 1990). It seems difficult to relate the apparent lack of adverse effects of zopiclone on the sleep profile to its biochemical action on a specific benzodiazepine-receptor subtype because it is well established that triazolam, an effective and potent sedative-hypnotic triazolobenzodiazepine, depresses REM sleep and yet appears to occupy a similar binding site on the benzodiazepine receptor as zopiclone (Chweh et al., 1985). This serves to emphasize the caution that must be exercised in extrapolating from in vitro experiments in the animal brain to in vivo studies in man.

In animal studies, the cyclopyrrolone suriclone has been shown to have a profile that is essentially similar to the 'classical' benzodiazepines in that it has an anti-aggressive effect in male mice, has a typical anxiolytic profile in the elevate plus maze and Geller–Seifter conflict test at doses that do not apparently cause muscle relaxation or sedation. In man, suriclone has been demonstrated to be effective in its treatment of generalized anxiety disorder (Julou et al., 1985). It has also been shown to have a lower propensity to potentiate the sedative effects of alcohol in mice. This implies that suriclone may be associated with a lower incidence of vigilance impairment in man than is frequently found with the long half-life benzodiazepines.

Whether other effects may be ascribed to a selectivity of action on the benzodiazepine receptors is a matter of conjecture. It is possible that the more clinically desirable profile of the cyclopyrrolones is more a product of lower receptor occupancy, shorter half-life and lower receptor affinity compared with the 'classical' benzodiazepines than any fundamental difference in the way in which they modulate the benzodiazepine–GABA receptor complex.

Faull and co-workers (1987) reported that the experimental triazolopyridazine compound Cl 218.872 displaced ³H-diazepam, and had a much greater affinity for cerebellar than for hippocampal or cortical membranes in human brain. These findings indicated that sites labelled by the benzodiazepines are heterogenous. Furthermore, such differences in receptor specificity might account for the pharmacological effects of Cl 128.872. This compound was shown to be anxiolytic, which in the absence of sedation in animal tests led to the hypothesis that this cerebellar benzodiazepine receptor subtype (the Bz1 type) is responsible for the anxiolytic effect of the benzodiazepines while the other type of receptor found in the higher centres of the brain (the Bz2 type) is associated with muscle relaxation and sedation. The imidazopyridines, such as alpidem and zolpidem, were shown to have a higher affinity for the Bz1 type of receptor. Further studies showed that these drugs had a higher affinity for GABA-A receptors that contained α-1 subunits than those containing α-3 subunits in contrast with the 'classical' benzodiazepines that failed to discriminate between either the Bz1 or Bz2 receptor subtypes or GABA receptors that contained different proportions of α, β or γ subunits (Langer et al., 1992). Further experimental studies of zolpidem and alpidem led to the hypothesis that the anxiolytic and sedative effects were mediated by activation of the Bz1 receptors: those drugs that had a high intrinsic activity being sedative, whereas those with a low intrinsic activity were anxiolytic with a low sedative propensity. Alpidem was shown to be a partial agonist in Bz1 receptor studies, while zolpidem was a potent full agonist at these sites (Zivkovic et al., 1992). This led to the classification of alpidem as a novel anxiolytic and zolpidem as a sedative–hypnotic. In experimental studies, these imidazopyridines are virtually devoid of muscle relaxant activity and have a low potential to cause amnesia (Zivkovic et al., 1990). Tolerance and physical dependence have been reported not to occur in animals (Perrault et al., 1992) or man (Chevalier et al., 1993). Whether more detailed experimental and clinical studies will confirm these initial findings remains to be established. If confirmed, it remains to be explained why benzodiazepine-receptor ligands that selectively activate Bz1 receptors that are located primarily in the cerebellum act as specific anxiolytics and sedative–hypnotics. Convention would predict that those areas of the brain subserving anxiety and vigilance are the hippocampus and locus coeruleus that contain predominately Bz2 receptors. Is it possible that the functional differences among the imidazopyridines are more related to the different densities of benzodiazepine–GABA-A receptors and their degree of occupancy in the relevant brain regions? (Haefely *et al.*, 1992). Such a 'receptor-reserve' hypothesis is based on the observation that the pharmacological effects of the 'classical' benzodiazepines vary according to the dose of drug administered. For example, the anxiolytic effects of diazepam occur at lower doses than the sedative effects while relatively high therapeutic doses of the drug are necessary to cause muscle relaxation. By definition, partial agonists at the benzodiazepine-receptor site (e.g. bretazenil or alpidem) would not cause sedation or muscle relaxation even at their highest concentrations. Thus, only a fraction of all the receptors need to be occupied by a full agonist to achieve a desired effect (e.g. sedation) and the remaining receptors constitute the receptor reserve. If such 'spare' receptors are occupied, then other pharmacological effects such as muscle relaxation occur. In short, the receptor occupancy necessary for a specific pharmacological effect is inversely related to the efficacy of the ligand and those ligands with low efficacy may not reach the level of receptor occupancy necessary to result in such undesirable side effects as muscle relaxation.

In an attempt to develop anxiolytics that lack the sedative, muscle relaxant and amnesic properties of the full benzodiazepine agonists such as diazepam, attention has been directed towards the beta-carbolines. Abercarnil is now undergoing clinical development as an anxiolytic with anticonvulsant properties without the unacceptable side effects of the conventional benzodiazepines (Spencer and Benfield, 1995). Abercarnil is a beta-carboline which acts as a partial benzodiazepine agonist. Experimental studies have shown that this drug has a greater affinity for the Bz2 receptors than diazepam and, in experimental studies, shows all the characteristics of a partial agonist at benzodiazepine receptors (Spencer and Benfield, 1995). In addition, abercarnil has been shown to produce anxiolytic activity at receptor occupancies lower (about 50%) than those required by diazepam to exert the same anxiolytic effects. Such a profile more closely reflects that of a full agonist at benzodiazepine receptors than a partial agonist and suggests that abercarnil may act as a full agonist at some benzodiazepine receptors but a partial agonist at others. Experimental studies have also shown that abercarnil has a lower dependence-producing potential than conventional full agonists at benzodiazepine receptors and shows a lower abuse potential and a lower alcohol potentiation than drugs such as diazepam. Despite the interesting experimental studies, so far there is only very limited clinical data available. In a placebo-controlled trial of abercarnil in generalized anxiety disorder, low doses (3–9 mg/day) were more effective than placebo and had fewer side effects than diazepam. Higher doses (7.5–30 mg/day) produced typical benzodiazepine-like adverse effects and some withdrawal effects were reported (Ballenger *et al.*, 1991). Clearly, more detailed clinical trials, particularly in the lower dose range, will be necessary before any conclusion may be made regarding the superiority of this beta-carboline in the treatment of anxiety disorders.

CONCLUSIONS

Despite the dependence-producing effects of the conventional benzodiazepines, the conventional 1,4-benzodiazepines continue to be widely used as anxiolytics and sedative–hypnotics. Knowledge of the nature of the benzodiazepine receptor and its relationship with the GABA-A receptor has illustrated the richness of the pharmacology based on the diazepine structure. While this has resulted in the development of full agonists, apart from the partial agonist clobazam and its desmethyl metabolite, no other therapeutic agents have been developed to date. Perhaps it is timely for the pharmaceutical industry to consider such developments.

REFERENCES

Ballenger, J.C., McDonald, S., Noyes, R. *et al.* (1991). The first double-blind trials of the partial benzodiazepine agonist abercarnil (2K-112-119) in generalized anxiety disorder. *Psychopharmacol Bull* **27**, 171–177.

Beaumont, G. (1995). Clobazam in the treatment of anxiety. *Hum Psychopharmacol* **10**, S27–S41.

Benke, D., Mertens, S., Trzeciak, A., Gillessen, D. and Mohler, H. (1991). GABA-A receptors display association of gamma 2-subunit with alpha-1 and beta-2/3 subunits. *J Biol Chem* **226**, 4478–4483.

Bowery, N. (1989). GABA-B receptors and their significance in mammalian pharmacology. *Trends Pharmacol Sci* **10**, 401–407.

Bowery, N. (1993). Aspects of the molecular pharmacology of GABA-B receptors. *Ann Rev Pharmacol Toxicol* **33**, 109–147.

Braestrup, C. and Nielsen, M. (1983). Benzodiazepine receptors. In: Iversen, L.L., Iversen, S.D. and Snyder, S.H. (Eds), *Handbook of Psychopharmacology*. Plenum Press, New York, pp. 285–384.

Braestrup, C. and Squires, R.F. (1978). No change in rat benzodiazepine receptors after withdrawal from continuous treatment with lorazepam and diazepam. *Life Sci* **24**, 347–350.

Chevalier, J.F., Mendlewicz, J., Coupez, R. and Garreau, M. (1993). Safety and efficacy of alpidem: long-term open-label observations. In: Bartholini, G., Garreau, M., Morselli, P.L. and Zivkovic, B. (Eds), *Imidazopyridines in Anxiety Disorders*. Raven Press, New York, pp. 183–192.

Chweh, A.Y., Swinyard, E.A. and Wolf, H.H. (1985). Gamma-amino butyric acid: temperature dependence in benzodiazepine receptor binding. *J Neurochem* **45**, 240–243.

Collins, P., Sakalis, G. and Minn, F.L. (1976). Clinical response to a potential non-sedative anxiolytic. *Curr Therapeut Res* **19**, 513–515.

Cook, L. and Stepinwall, J. (1995). Behavioural analysis of the effects and mechanisms of action of benzodiazepines. *Adv Biochem Psychopharmacol* **14**, 1–28.

Costa, E., Guildotti, A., Mao, C.C. and Suria, A. (1975). New concepts on the mechanism of action of benzodiazepines. *Life Sci* **17**, 167–186.

Delini-Stula, A. (1992). Bretazenil: clinical experience. *Neurosci Facts* **3**, 72.

Facklam, M., Schoch, P., Bonetti, E.P., Jenck, F., Martin, J.R., Moreau, J. and Haefely, W.E. (1992). Relationship between benzodiazepine receptor occupancy and functional effects in vivo of four ligands of differing intrinsic efficacies. *J Pharmacol Exp Ther* **261**, 1113–21.

Faull, R.L., Villiger, J.W. and Holford, N.H. (1987). Benzodiazepine receptors in the human cerebellar cortex: a quantative autoradiographic and pharmacological study demonstrating the predominance of type I receptors. *Brain Res* **411**, 317–385.

Fielding, S. and Hoffman, I. (1979). Pharmacology of anti-anxiety drugs with special reference to clobazam. *Br J Clin Pharmacol* **7**, 7S–15S.

Haefely, W. (1990). Benzodiazepine receptors and ligands: structural and functional differences. In: Hindmarch, I., Beaumont, G., Brandon, S. and Leonard, B.E. (Eds), *Benzodiazepines Current Concepts*. Chichester: John Wiley and Sons, pp. 1–18.

Haefely, W., Kulcsar, A., Moehler, H., Pieri, L., Polc, P. and Schaffner, R. (1975). Possible involvement in GABA in the central actions of benzodiazepines. In: Costa, E. and Greengard, P. (Eds), *Mechanism of Action of Benzodiazepines*. Raven Press, New York, pp. 131–152.

Haefely, W., Kyburz, E., Gerecke, M. and Moehler, H. (1985). Recent advances in the molecular pharmacology of benzodiazepine receptors and in the structure–activity relationship of their agonists and antagonists. *Adv Drug Res* **124**, 165–322.

Haefely, W., Martin, J.R. and Schoch, P. (1990). Novel anxiolytics acting as partial agonists at benzodiazepine receptors. *Trends Pharmacol Sci* **11**, 452–456.

Haefely, W., Bonetti, E.P., Facklam, M. *et al.* (1992). Partial agonists of benzodiazepine receptors for the treatment of epilepsy, sleep and anxiety disorders. *Adv Biochem Psychopharmacol* **47**, 379–394.

Hindmarch, I. (1995). The psychopharmacology of clobazam. *Hum Psychopharmacol* **10**, S15–S25.

Johnson, G. (1991). GABA-A antagonists. *Semin Neurosci* **3**, 205–210.

Julou, L., Bardone, M.C.C. and Blanchard, J.C. (1983). Pharmacological studies on zopiclone. *Pharmacology* **27**, 46–58.

Julou, L., Blanchard, J.C. and Preyfus, J.F. (1985). Pharmacological and clinical studies of cyclopyrrolones: zopiclone and suriclone. *Pharmacol Biochem Behav* **23**, 653–659.

Koeppen, D. (1985). A review of clobazam studies in epilepsy. In: Hindmarch, I., Stonier, P.D. and Trimble, M. (Eds), *Clobazam: Human Psychopharmacology and Clinical Applications*. International Congress and Symposium Series, No. 74. The Royal Society of Medicine, London, pp. 207–215.

Langer, S.A., Faure-Halley, C., Seeburg, F., Graham, D. and Arbilla, S. (1992). The selectivity of zolpidem and alpidem for the alpha-1 subunit of the GABA-A receptor. *Eur Neuropsychopharmacol* **2**, 232–234.

Leonard, B.E. (1993). Commentary on the mode of action of benzodiazepines. *J Psychiatr Res* **27** (suppl 1), 193–207.

Lopez, F., Miller, G., Greenblatt, D.J., Chesley, S., Schatzki, A. and Shader, R.I. (1990). Chronic administration of benzodiazepines. V. Rapid onset of behavioural and neurochemical alterations after discontinuation of alprazolam. *Neuropharmacology* **29**, 237–241.

Malizia, A.A. and Nutt, D.J. (1995). Psychopharmacology of benzodiazepines – an update. *Hum Psychopharmacol* **10**, S1–S14.

Mandenna, J.S., Swanson, L.M., Dios-Vietez, M.C., Hollander-Jansen, M. and Danhof, M. (1991). Pharmacokinetic-pharmacodynamic modeling of the electro-cephalographic effects of benzodiazepines. Correction with receptor binding and anti-convulsant activity. *J Pharmacol Exp Ther* **257**, 472–478.

Mohler, H. and Fritschy, J.M. (1992). Expression of GABA-A receptor subtypes. *Neurosci Facts* **3**, 70–71.

Mohler, H. and Okada, T. (1977). Benzodiazepine receptor: demonstration in the central nervous system. *Science* **198**, 849–851.

Mohler, H., Malherse, P., Draguan, A. *et al.* (1990). GABA receptors: structural requirements and sites of gene expression in mammalian brain. *Neurochem Res* **15**, 199–207.

Musch, B. and Maillard, F. (1990). Zopiclone, the third generation hypnotic: a clinical overview. *Int Clin Psychopharmacol* **5**(suppl 2), 147–158.

Noggin, T. and Callaghan, N. (1985). Blood levels of clobazam and its metabolites and therapeutic effects. In: Hindmarch, I., Stonier, P.D. and Trimble, M. (Eds), *Clobazam: Human Psychopharmacology and Clinical Applications*. International Congress and Symposium Series, No. 74. The Royal Society of Medicine, London, pp. 149–154.

Olsen, R.W. and Venter, C.J. (Eds) (1980). *Benzodiazepine–GABA Receptors and Chloride Channels: Structural and Functional Properties*. Alan R. Liss, New York.

Perrault, G., Morel, E., Sanger, D.J. and Zivkovic, B. (1992). Lack of tolerance and physical dependence upon repeated treatment with the novel hypnotic zolpidem. *J Pharmacol Exp Ther* **236**, 298–303.

Polc, P. and Haefely, W. (1977). Effects of system muscimol and GMBA in the spinal cord and superior cervical ganglion in the cat. *Experienta* **33**, 809–813.

Polc, P., Mohler, H. and Haefely, W. (1974). The effect of diazepam and spinal cord activities: possible sites and mechanisms of action. *Naunyn Schmiedebergs Arch Pharmacol* **284**, 319–337.

Potier, M.C., Prado de Carallo, L., Dodd, R.H., Brown, C.C. and Rosier, J. (1988). *In vivo* binding of [3]H R 15-1788 in mice: comparison with the *in vivo* binding of ^{3}H-flumitrazepam. *Life Sci* **43**, 1287–1296.

Richards, G., Schoch, P. and Haefely, W. (1991). Benzodiazepine receptors: new vistas. *Semin Neurosci* **3**, 191–203.

Robertson, MM. (1995). The place of clobazam in the treatment of epilepsy: an update. *Hum Psychopharmacol* **10**, S43–S63.

Spencer, C.M. and Benfield, P. (1995). Abercarnil in generalized anxiety disorder. *CNS Drugs* **3**, 69–82.

Squires, R.F. and Braestrup, C. (1977). Benzodiazepine receptors in rat brain. *Nature* **266**, 732–734.

Sternbach, L.H. (1983). The discovery of CNS active 1,4-benzodiazepines. In: Costa, E. (Ed.), *The Benzodiazepines: From Biology to Clinical Practice*. Raven Press, New York, pp. 1–6.

Sternbach, L.H., Randall, L.O., Banziger, R. and Lehr, H. (1986). Structure–activity relationships in the 1,4-benzodiazepine series. In: Burger, A. (Ed.), *Drugs affecting the Central Nervous System*. Marcel Dekker, New York, pp. 237–264.

Tallman, J.F. and Gallagher, D.W. (1985). The GABA-ergic system: a locus of benzo-diazepine action. *Ann Rev Neurosci* **8**, 21–44.

Ticku, M.K. (1991). Drug modulation of GABA-A mediated transmission. *Semin Neurosci* **3**, 211–219.

Trifiletti, R.R. and Snyder, S.H. (1984). Anxiolytic cyclopyrrolones zopiclone and suriclone bind to a novel site linked allosterically to benzodiazepine receptors. *Mol Pharmacol* **26**, 456–458.

Van der Meyen, C.H., Bartel, P.R., Somers, D.E.K., Bloom, M. and Pretorius, L.C. (1989). Effects of clobazam and clonazepam on saccadic eye movements and the parameters of psychomotor performance. *Eur J Clin Pharmacol* **37**, 365–369.

Volz, M., Christ, O., Kellner, M.M. *et al.* (1979). Kinetics and metabolism of clobazam in animals and man. *Br J Clin Pharmacol* **7**, 41S–50S.

Zivkovic, B., Morel, E., Jolly, D., Perrault, G., Sanger, D.J. and Lloyd, K.G. (1990). Pharmacological and behavioural profile of alpidem as an anxiolytic. *Pharmacopsychiatry* **23**, 108–113.

Zivkovic, B., Perrault, G. and Sanger, D.J. (1992). Receptor subtype selective drugs: a new generation of anxiolytics and hypnotics. In: Mendlewicz, J. and Racagnni, G. (Eds), *Target Receptors for Anxiolytics and Hypnotics from Molecular Pharmacology to Therapeutics.* Karger, Basel, pp. 55–73.

2

Benzodiazepines, Memory and Cognitive Function

H. VALERIE CURRAN

Clinical Health Psychology, University College London, London, UK

INTRODUCTION

Many centrally acting drugs affect 'cognitive function' – the way in which past knowledge is used to interpret and act upon current experience. Clinically, understanding the adverse cognitive effects of a prescribed psychotropic is as important as understanding its adverse physical effects. For patients who take drugs on a regular basis, a drug treatment that impairs memory or concentration could interfere significantly with their ability to work, study or cope with the general cognitive demands of daily living.

The cognitive effects of the benzodiazepines have probably been studied in greater detail than any other drugs in history. A central focus has been on the memory impairments produced by these drugs. A single dose of a benzodiazepine induces a temporary anterograde amnesia. This property of benzodiazepines has been viewed positively by anaesthetists who have administered these drugs as premedicants since the early 1960s. The fact that patients remember little if anything of their subsequent experiences during surgery is seen as a very desirable effect of the benzodiazepines. What is positive for an anaesthetist, however, is negative for the patient who takes these drugs regularly for anxiety disorders or sleep problems. Ghoneim and Mewaldt (1990) point out that the marketing of these drugs by pharmaceutical companies led to some inconsistencies in the information given to doctors: *The Physician's Handbook* in 1989 promoted intravenous Valium (diazepam) to anaesthetists on the basis of its remarkable ability to induce total amnesia in patients; a few chapters later, the very same drug given orally is promoted as a daily treatment for anxiety disorders with no mention of any effect it may have on memory.

The vast majority of studies on the benzodiazepines and cognition have assessed the effects of single doses in healthy volunteers and this research is summarized in the next section. The degree to which apparent memory effects of benzodiazepines might relate to their other cognitive effects or to their sedative effects is also examined. There is a relative paucity of research on patients who take these drugs regularly and this literature is overviewed in the following section.

Finally, the importance of assessing the memory effects of new drug treatments is discussed in terms of the types of assessments used and the populations tested.

BENZODIAZEPINES AND MEMORY

Memory is central to cognitive functions, and is involved in almost all our information processing. However, 'memory' is an umbrella term which covers a range of different processes and systems. For example, 'memory' for the skills of driving a car is distinguishable from 'memory' for a recent visit to the theatre or from 'memory' for a telephone number you might store temporarily while dialling. Studies with brain-damaged people have shown that these different kinds of memory are neurobiologically separable. Similarly, pharmacological studies have shown dissociations between drug effects on different aspects of memory.

Specific benzodiazepine receptors are found in greatest concentrations in brain areas that neuropsychologists have shown are critically involved in memory functions: the cerebral cortex, cerebellum and limbic system (including hippocampus and amygdala). It is therefore not surprising that benzodiazepines exert their most robust and marked cognitive effects upon human memory. The benzodiazepines have fascinated memory researchers because single doses of these drugs impair certain aspects of memory whilst sparing other aspects. Further, studies using benzodiazepines to induce a pharmacological amnesia have theoretical importance that complements research with brain-damaged people or research showing functional or developmental dissociations (Nyberg and Tulving, 1996).

Studies in healthy volunteers

Transient anterograde 'amnesia' is a consistent finding from volunteer studies of single doses of a benzodiazepine: information presented after the drug is administered is poorly remembered. In contrast, no study has found objective evidence of retrograde impairments of memory: information acquired before drug administration is retained intact. These drugs therefore impede the acquisition of new information. The degree and duration of anterograde amnesia following an acute dose depends on several factors: dosage and route of administration; the particular benzodiazepine taken; the memory assessments used; the times post-drug at which information is presented and retrieval is required; characteristics of the subject population tested. Although there is considerable variation between studies in these factors, the relatively large number of studies carried out to date allows some generalizations to be drawn out.

In general, benzodiazepines do not affect the performance of tasks that require remembering a few items for a period of seconds (e.g. digit span, block span). In more complex tasks where information needs to be manipulated whilst it is retained, benzodiazepine-induced deficits are often found. So impairments are found where higher cognitive effort is required, such as dividing attention between two simultaneous tasks. On the whole, the evidence points to a reduction in the speed with which information is processed rather than qualitative effects on components of executive function or working memory. For example, error rates are generally much less affected than response times (Curran, 1986; 1991).

The benzodiazepines affect different aspects of long-term memory in different ways. Memory theorists debate how best to characterize long-term remembering in terms of systems, processes and functions. A useful framework that most neatly encompasses drug effects is Tulving's 'memory systems' account (Tulving, 1985; Tulving and Schacter, 1990). This distinguishes between episodic, semantic, procedural and perceptual representational systems.

Episodic memory, as its name suggests, is concerned with remembering personally experienced episodes in our lives. It is an autobiographical memory which retains information such as what movie you last saw, when and where. Critically, it is memory accompanied by conscious awareness (what Tulving terms 'autonoetic consciousness'), which allows the rememberer to re-experience the episode in his or her mind. A consistent and robust finding across more than a hundred studies is that the benzodiazepines impair performance of tasks tapping episodic memory. This impairment is clearly dose-dependent. In general, the more demands a task places on episodic memory, the clearer are the detrimental effects of the benzodiazepines. So, for example, free recall tasks are more sensitive than cued recall or recognition tasks.

Overall, when direct or explicit assessments of memory are used, the experimental manipulations that affect the performance of normal (non-drugged) people produce a parallel pattern of influences on the performance of people given a benzodiazepine. Thus, if people are required to process information at different depths, from the relatively superficial (e.g. deciding whether a word is in capital letters or in lower case) to the relatively deep (e.g. deciding whether a word belongs to a particular semantic category), benzodiazepines will result in fewer words being recalled but the pattern of recall will be the same as normal (i.e. deeper levels of encoding lead to better recall) (Curran *et al.*, 1988; Bishop and Curran, 1995). Further, rehearsal effects are normal with benzodiazepines (Mewaldt *et al.*, 1983) as is the forgetting rate (Brown *et al.*, 1983).

Episodic memory retains not only information *per se*, but details of the context in which the information was acquired. For example, when you recall what you had for dinner two nights ago, you will also recall contextual details – who you were with, when, where you sat, perhaps the smell of the food cooking or of the wine you drank. It is this richness of encoding that allows us to travel through subjective time from the present to the past in our individual autobiographies. Deficits in the encoding of contextual information have been put forward as a possible mechanism for benzodiazepine-induced impairment of episodic memory (e.g. Brown and Brown, 1990). Often, people with organic amnesia show profound impairments in memory for context such that even if they do remember a person's face or a new fact, they cannot recall where they met that person or learnt that fact. Studies of the benzodiazepines have usually found that memory for context is impaired as well as memory for the central information (e.g. Gorissen *et al.*, 1998). One explanation of both effects is that benzodiazepines impair the acquisition or consolidation of new associations *per se*, whether this is between different events or between a single event and its context.

Retrieval of well-established (semantic) knowledge is generally intact following drug administration (cf. Ghoneim and Mewaldt, 1990; Polster, 1993). Tasks tapping semantic memory – our shared knowledge of the world – do not show benzodiazepine-induced impairments. For example, verbal fluency is unaffected by drugs and in sentence-verification tasks error rates are not increased although drugs often increase the time to complete the task. Further, conceptual priming in category-generation tasks is intact following benzodiazepines, even though the explicit recall of studied category exemplars by individuals is very poor (Bishop and Curran, 1998).

The contents of episodic and semantic memory are thought to be directly accessible to consciousness – it is possible to bring to mind both personal episodes and impersonal facts. In contrast, procedural memory is expressed indirectly through skilled performance. The benzodiazepines do not affect procedural learning in perceptual-learning tasks (e.g. mirror reading) or in anagram-solving tasks (e.g. Weingartner and Wolkovitz, 1988). In tasks that have a significant motor response component and/or where speed of reaction time is critical (e.g. pursuit rotor, serial reaction time), a drug effect may be found but this is usually a general slowing of performance related to the drug's sedative effect (e.g. Nissen *et al.*, 1987; Curran, 1991). Critically, learning curves on drugs tend to parallel those on placebo.

Tasks assessing procedural memory in these ways are indirect tests of memory – remembering is inferred from changes in the performance of a skill. Another kind of indirect or implicit test of memory includes what is usually termed 'priming': the influence of prior exposure on subsequent performance. In priming tasks, the participants are not asked explicitly to remember information. Instead, memory is gauged implicitly from alterations in performance following exposure to information.

As already noted, there is some evidence that conceptual priming is intact following the benzodiazepines, fitting the usual preservation of semantic memory. Perceptual priming is thought to depend on a different memory system – the perceptual representation system (PRS). In a typical perceptual priming task, participants might be asked to rate a series of words (e.g. CHEESE, TRUMPET) according to how much they like each word. They are then asked to do an ostensibly unrelated task of completing word stems (e.g. TRU..., CHE..., MEA...) with the first word that comes to mind. Perceptual priming is indexed by the greater number of stems completed with words previously rated than base rates. Using such tasks, one benzodiazepine, lorazepam, has been found to produce impairments whereas others (alprazolam, triazolam, diazepam, oxazepam, midazolam) do not. This is an intriguing dissociation given that the benzodiazepines as a class are chemically very similar, and all produce impairments on explicit memory tasks.

Originally noted by Brown and colleagues (1989), this effect of lorazepam on perceptual priming has been replicated by several groups of researchers (Knopman, 1991; Danion *et al.*, 1992; Curran and Gorenstein, 1993; Vidailhet *et al.*, 1994; Stewart *et al.*, 1996). Several studies have compared lorazepam directly with another benzodiazepine and shown that both produce similar impairment on explicit tasks but only lorazepam impaired perceptual priming (Sellal *et al.*, 1992; Legrand *et al.*, 1995; Bishop *et al.*, 1996). Using experimental manipulations in accordance with Schacter's retrieval intentionality criterion, it was found that lorazepam impaired word-stem completion and this effect was attenuated by co-administration of the benzodiazepine antagonist, flumazenil (Bishop and Curran, 1995). Taken together, these studies imply that there are qualitative differences among benzodiazepines in their effects on memory.

SPECIFICITY OF BENZODIAZEPINE AMNESIA

An ongoing debate in research in cognitive psychopharmacology of memory centres on the specificity of benzodiazepine effects on memory. At a pharmacological level, there is the question of the degree of overlap in the pattern of memory effects of benzodiazepines with drugs that have different pharmacological actions such as scopolamine. At a psychological level, there is the question of how much the drug's amnesic effects are by-products of its effects on arousal or attentional functions.

Benzodiazepines: attention and memory

It could be argued that benzodiazepines may reduce attentional resources and thereby impede encoding of information. Gorissen and Ehling (1998) carried out two experiments in which participants were given dual tasks. They performed a visual discrimination task of varying levels of complexity concurrently with a paired-associate learning task. The benzodiazepine diazepam (15 mg) impaired subsequent recall of paired associates, but the level of impairment did not interact with the level of complexity of the visual discrimination task. Although dividing attention did reduce people's memory performance, it was no more disruptive to those given diazepam than to those given placebo. This would suggest that reduced attentional resources cannot account for the amnesic effects of benzodiazepines.

Several other studies have shown dissociations between the effects of benzodiazepines on attentional and memory functions. For example, Smirne and colleagues (1989) compared three dose levels of flunitrazepam (1, 2 and 4 mg) and found memory impairments even at the lowest dose, whereas accompanying attentional impairments were produced only by the higher doses. Or again, Hommer *et al.* (1993) administered the antagonist before giving diazepam and this resulted in a blocking of attentional and sedative effects but amnesia remained. Coull and colleagues (1995) compared the attentional effects of a range of drugs, including diazepam, and obtained differential effects.

Benzodiazepines: memory and sedation

Are the amnesic effects of the benzodiazepines wholly or partly by-products of the sedative effects of the benzodiazepines? One way of dissociating sedative effects from specific amnesic effects would be to show that different drugs may produce the same effects on sedation but different effects on memory or vice versa. For example, the effects of three different drugs were compared with placebo: the benzodiazepine lorazepam (2 mg by mouth), the sedative antihistamine diphenhydramine (25, 50 mg by mouth) and the anticholinergic drug scopolamine (0.6 mg subcutaneously) (Curran *et al.*, 1998). The 50 mg dose of the antihistamine produced similar levels of sedation to scopolamine and lorazepam. However, unlike scopolamine and the benzodiazepine, it did not impair performance on a task tapping episodic memory. Event-related potentials (ERPs) recorded simultaneously showed that earlier components were affected similarly by all three drugs whereas later components such as P_{300} were more affected by scopolamine and lorazepam than by the antihistamine. This study therefore provides evidence that the amnesic effects of the benzodiazepines are dissociated from their sedative effects.

Evidence from other kinds of dissociations supports this conclusion. For instance, differential dose–response curves on measures of memory and sedation were demonstrated in the study by Weingartner and colleagues (1993) of three doses of triazolam. Another type of dissociation would be to show differential reversal of amnesic and sedative effects by a benzodiazepine antagonist such as flumazenil. Studies with flumazenil have produced an inconsistent pattern of results because different studies have used different agonist/antagonist dosages. Complete reversal of amnesic effects by flumazenil has sometimes been reported (Dorow *et al.*, 1987; Gentil *et al.*, 1989). Ghoneim and colleagues (1989) found that the time course of flumazenil's reversal of diazepam's effects differed for sedation compared with amnesia. Reversal of sedative and psychomotor effects of midazolam but not its amnesic effects has also been found (Birch and Curran, 1990; Curran and Birch, 1991). A fair conclusion is probably that sedative and attentional effects are more easily reversed, and at lower antagonist doses, than amnesic effects. Many other studies have covaried measures of sedation from measures of memory and found that significant drug impairments in memory remain. Taken as a whole, the various approaches to differentiating sedation and amnesia support the notion that the benzodiazepines have specific amnesic effects over and above their sedative effects. Research with anxious patients, discussed below, also supports this conclusion.

Studies of repeated doses of benzodiazepines

Studies of the memory and cognitive effects of single doses of benzodiazepines clearly cannot be generalized to patients who take drugs on a repeated basis for anxiety disorders or insomnia. Tolerance develops to benzodiazepines, although at different rates to different effects. For example, Ghoneim and colleagues (1981) showed that volunteers given diazepam daily for 3 weeks developed tolerance to drug effects on immediate but not delayed (15 min) recall of a word list. Morton and Lader (1992) assessed patients diagnosed with generalized anxiety disorder before and after a 4-week treatment with either lorazepam (mean end of treatment dose, 1.7 mg b.d.) or alpidem (mean end of treatment dose 56 mg b.d.). Both treatments produced parallel reductions in anxiety levels and at 4 weeks there was no subjective or motor sedation. However, patients given lorazepam were significantly impaired on a word recall task at 4 weeks. Thus, tolerance had developed to sedative but not anxiolytic or amnesic effects of lorazepam. In a study of long-term (> 6 months) users of benzodiazepines, Golombok and colleagues (1988) found that a measure of the cumulative intake of benzodiazepines correlated negatively with level of learning in word recall task trials, as too did the actual dose of benzodiazepine taken on the day of assessment.

There has been one randomized controlled trial that compared the effects of the benzodiazepine alprazolam with placebo in 38 agoraphobia/panic patients (Curran *et al.*, 1994). Significant and marked impairments on word recall were found after 8 weeks of treatment with alprazolam. Reassessment of patients at 24 weeks, when they had been free of medication for 5–8 weeks, showed that alprazolam patients were still impaired on recall compared with placebo patients. However, these impairments did not persist at a long-term follow-up 3.5 years later (Cilic *et al.*, 1999). In a study of benzodiazepine withdrawal, Tata and colleagues (1994) assessed 21 patients taking benzodiazepines on a long-term basis (average of 13 years) at three time points: whilst on medication, 10 days after their last dose and again 6 months later. Compared with normal controls, patients showed little improvement between the first and second testing. Patients were particularly impaired on verbal memory tasks and on a task tapping visuo-motor and attentional capacities. At 6 months follow-up, patients performed less well than controls and showed little improvement since their initial testing. Further, the dose of diazepam that they had taken correlated significantly with the degree of cognitive deficit observed 6 months following withdrawal.

The findings of Curran and colleagues (1994) and Tata and colleagues (1994) imply that benzodiazepines block the improvement in performance that normally accompanies practice of cognitive tasks. These studies did not find impairments on simple psychomotor tasks which are sensitive to the sedative effects of a single dose of a benzodiazepine. Thus, they also imply that tolerance over repeated dosing builds up differentially such that patients may not notice sedative effects after a time period but may experience a degree of memory impairment for many years. The time course for recovery of function when patients stop chronic use of benzodiazepines is not clear from published studies, but may be between 6 months (follow-up period of Tata and colleagues) and 3.5 years (follow-up period of Curran and colleagues).

CONCLUSIONS

The importance of testing the effects of novel drug treatments on memory and cognition is emphasized by the history of research on benzodiazepines. Although research on single doses of new compounds in volunteers would be a relevant starting point, studies also need to be carried out with patients who take medication over a normal treatment period.

Partly due to pharmacokinetic changes with age, older people can be particularly sensitive to drug-induced memory impairment. Older people are sometimes prescribed several psychoactive drugs, and this may cause a drug-induced 'pseudo-dementia', with confusion and memory loss sharing similarities with organic dementia. In Europe, people over 65 years old are the major consumers of hypnotics – both the benzodiazepines and the newer compounds such as zopiclone, which have similar effects on gamma-aminobutyric acid (GABA). Salzman and colleagues (1992) demonstrated improved memory in older people who withdrew from daily benzodiazepine use compared with those who were maintained on benzodiazepines. It is lamentable that people in these age groups are so often excluded from clinical trials, especially as they constitute a rapidly increasing proportion of the world's population.

A comment is also warranted on the tests used to assess memory and cognition. These need to be selected in order to sample the full range of systems known as memory, attention and executive function. Further, there is often too much reliance on artificial laboratory tests, which may say little about how a drug affects a patient's daily cognitive function. There are tests that have more ecological validity and sample the demands of everyday life, and these should be incorporated into clinical trials.

The use of radiolabelled drugs in imaging studies is already allowing delineation of receptors in the living brain, and this will provide a means of assessing abnormalities in psychiatric and neurological disorders. A drug and placebo can also be administered during functional imaging and this allows drug-induced changes in activation to be monitored during performance of a memory task (cf. Fletcher *et al.*, 1996). Such refinements in the techniques for studying the effects of drugs will have important clinical repercussions for the development of new drug treatments.

REFERENCES

Birch, B. and Curran, H.V. (1990). The differential effects of flumazenil on the psychomotor and amnesic actions of midazolam. *J Psychopharmacol* **4**, 29–34.

Bishop, B. and Curran, H.V. (1995). Psychopharmacological analysis of implicit and explicit memory: a study with lorazepam and the benzodiazepine antagonist, flumazenil. *Psychopharmacology* **121**, 267–278.

Bishop, K. and Curran, H.V. (1998). An investigation of the effects of benzodiazepine receptor ligands and of scopolamine on conceptual priming. *Psychopharmacology* **140**, 345–353.

Bishop, K.I., Curran, H.V. and Lader, M. (1996). Do scopolamine and lorazepam have dissociable effects on human memory systems? A dose–response study with normal volunteers. *Exp Clin Psychopharmacol* **4**, 292–299.

Brown, J. and Brown, M.W. (1990). The effects of repeating a recognition test on lorazepam-induced amnesia: evidence for impaired contextual memory as a cause of amnesia. *Q J Exp Psychol* **42A**, 279–290.

Brown, J., Lewis, V., Brown, M.W., Horn, G. and Bowes, J.B. (1983). A comparison between transient amnesias induced by two drugs (diazepam and lorazepam) and amnesia of organic origin. *Neuropsychologia* **20**, 55–70.

Brown, M.W., Brown, J. and Bowes, J. (1989). Absence of priming coupled with substantially preserved recognition in lorazepam induced amnesia. *Q J Exp Psychol* **41A**, 599–617.

Cilic, G., Curran, H.V. and Marks, I. (1999). A four year follow-up of agoraphobia with panic disorder: lack of residual effects of alprazolam on memory. *Psychol Med* **29**, 225–231.

Coull, J.T., Sahakian, B.J., Middleton, H.C. *et al.* (1995). Differential effects of clonidine, haloperidol, diazepam and tryptophan depletion on focussed attention and attentional search. *Psychopharmacology* **121**, 222–230.

Curran, H.V. (1986). Tranquillizing memories: a review of the effects of benzodiazepines on human memory. *Biol Psychol* **23**, 179–213.

Curran, H.V. (1991). Benzodiazepines, memory and mood: a review. *Psychopharmacology* **105**, 1–8.

Curran, H.V. and Birch, B. (1991). Differentiating the sedative and amnestic effects of benzodiazepines: a study with midazolam and the benzodiazepine antagonist, flumazenil. *Psychopharmacology* **103**, 519–523.

Curran, H.V. and Gorenstein, C. (1993). Differential effects of lorazepam and oxazepam on priming. *Int Clin Psychopharmacol* **8**, 37–42.

Curran, H.V., Schiwy, W., Eves, F., Shine, P. and Lader, M.H. (1988). A 'levels of processing' study of the effects of benzodiazepines on human memory. *Hum Psychopharmacol* **3**, 21–25.

Curran, H.V., Bond, A., O'Sullivan, G. *et al.* (1994). Memory functions, alprazolam and exposure therapy: a controlled longitudinal study of patients with agoraphobia and panic disorder. *Psychol Med* **24**, 969–976.

Curran, H.V., Poovibunsuk, P., Dalton, J. and Lader, M.H. (1998). Differentiating the effects of centrally acting drugs on arousal and memory: an event-related potential study of scopolamine, lorazepam and diphenhydramine. *Psychopharmacology* **135**, 27–36.

Danion, J.M. Peretti, S. and Grange, D. (1992). Effects of chlorpromazine and lorazepam on explicit memory, repetition priming and cognitive skill learning in healthy volunteers. *Psychopharmacology* **108**, 345–351.

Dorow, R., Berenberg, D., Duka, T. and Sauergrey, N. (1987). Amnestic effects of lormetazepam and their reversal by the benzodiazepine antagonist Ro 15-1788. *Psychopharmacology* **93**, 507–514.

Fletcher, P.C., Frith, C.D., Grasby, P.M., Friston, K.J. and Dolan, R.I. (1996). Local and distributed effects of apomorphine on fronto-temporal function in acute unmedicated schizophrenics. *J Neurosci* **16**, 7055–7062.

Gentil, V., Tavares, S., Gorenstein, C. *et al.* (1989). Acute reversal of flunitrazepam effects by Ro 15-1788 and Ro 153505: inverse antagonism, tolerance, and rebound. *Psychopharmacology* **100**, 54–59.

Ghoneim, M.M. and Mewaldt, S.P. (1990). Benzodiazepines and human memory: a review. *Anesthesiology* **72**, 926–938.

Ghoneim, M.M., Mewaldt, S.P., Berie, J.L. and Hinrichs, V. (1981). Memory and performance effects of single and 3 week administration of diazepam. *Psychopharmacology* **73**, 147–151.

Ghoneim, M.M., Dembo, J.B. and Block, R.I. (1989). Time course of antagonism of sedative and amnesic effects of diazepam by flumazenil. *Anesthesiology* **70**, 899–904.

Golombok, S., Moodley, P. and Lader, M. (1988). Cognitive impairment in long-term benzodiazepine users. *Psychol Med* **18**, 365–374.

Gorissen, M.E.E. and Ehling, P.A.T.M. (1998). Dual task performance after diazepam intake: can resource depletion explain the benzodiazepine-induced amnesia? *Psychopharmacology* **138**, 354–361.

Gorissen, M.E.E., Curran, H.V. and Eling, P.A. (1998). Proactive interference and temporal context encoding after diazepam intake. *Psychopharmacology* **138**, 334–343.

Hommer, D., Weingartner, H.J. and Brier, A. (1993). Dissociation of benzodiazepine induced amnesia from sedation. *Psychopharmacology* **112**, 455–460.

Knopman, D. (1991). Unaware learning versus preserved learning in pharmacologic amnesia: similarities and differences. *J Exp Psychol Learn Mem Cogn* **17**, 1017–1029.

Legrand, F., Vidailhet, P., Danion, J.-M. *et al.* (1995). Time course of the effects of diazepam and lorazepam on perceptual priming and explicit memory. *Psychopharmacology* **118**, 475–479.

Mewaldt, S.P., Hinrichs, J.V. and Ghoneim, M.M. (1983). Diazepam and memory: support for a duplex model of memory. *Mem Cogn* **II**, 557–564.

Morton, S. and Lader, M.H. (1992). Alpidem and lorazepam in the treatment of patients with anxiety disorders: comparison of physiological and psychological effects. *Pharmacopsychiatry* **25**, 177–181.

Nissen, M.J., Knopman, D.S. and Schacter, D.L. (1987). Neurochemical dissociations of memory systems. *Neurology* **37**, 789–794.

Nyberg, L. and Tulving, E. (1996). Classifying human long-term memory: evidence from converging dissociations. *Eur J Cogn Psychol* **8**, 163–183.

Polster, M.R. (1993). Drug-induced amnesia: implications for cognitive neuropsychological investigations of memory. *Psychol Bull* **114**, 477–493.

Saltzman, C., Fisher, J., Nobel, K. *et al.* Cognitive improvement following benzodiazepine discontinuation in elderly nursing home residents. (1992). *Int J Geriatr Psychiatry* **7**, 89–93.

Sellal, F., Danion, J.M., Kauffmann-Mueller, F. *et al.* (1992). Differential effects of diazepam and lorazepam on repetition priming in healthy volunteers. *Psychopharmacology* **108**, 371–379.

Smirne, S., Ferini-Stambi, L., Pirola, R. *et al.* (1989). Effects of flunitrazepam on cognitive functions. *Psychopharmacology* **98**, 251–256.

Stewart, S.H., Rioux, G.F., Connolly, J.F., Dunphy, S.C. and Teehan, M.D. (1996). Effects of oxazepam and lorazepam on implicit and explicit memory: evidence for possible influences of time course. *Psychopharmacology* **128**, 139–149.

Tata, P.R., Rollings, J., Collins, M., Pickering, A. and Jacobsen, R.R. (1994). Lack of cognitive recovery following withdrawal from long-term benzodiazepine use. *Psychol Med* **24**, 203–213.

Tulving, E. (1985). How many memory systems are there? *Am Psychol* **40**, 385–398.

Tulving, E. and Schacter, D.L. (1990). Priming and human memory systems. *Science* **247**, 301–306.

Vidailhet, P., Danion, J.M., Kauffman-Muller, F. *et al.* (1994). Lorazepam and diazepam effects on memory acquisition in priming tests. *Psychopharmacology* **115**, 397–406.

Weingartner, H.J. and Wolkovitz, O. (1988). Pharmacological strategies for exploring the psychobiologically distinct cognitive systems. *Psychopharmacology* **S125**, 31–37.

Weingartner, H.J., Joyce, E.M., Sirocco, K.Y. *et al.* (1993). Specific memory and sedative effects of the benzodiazepine triazolam. *J Psychopharmacol* **7**, 305–315.

Benzodiazepines
Edited by Michael R. Trimble and Ian Hindmarch
© 2000 Wrightson Biomedical Publishing Ltd

3

Management of Sleep Disorders in Primary Care

GEORGE BEAUMONT

Visiting Professor, HPRU, University of Surrey, Guildford, UK

INTRODUCTION

Difficulty sleeping is a common problem. In addition to the concern that disturbed sleep generates, the daytime drowsiness that insomnia and other causes of lack of sleep lead to, is a major public health issue. The majority of complaints of poor sleep are presented and dealt with in primary care.

Studies undertaken in the USA suggest that as many as 30% of the population has some difficulty in falling asleep or maintaining sleep and that 17% of individuals affected perceive this as serious (Mellinger *et al.*, 1985). Similar figures have been found in studies undertaken elsewhere in the world, including a UK study (Mniszek, 1988).

It has been estimated that nearly four out of ten individuals do not get a good night's sleep (Mellinger *et al.*, 1985) and, as a consequence, function during the day at an impaired level of alertness. Amongst elderly people it has been estimated that as many as 60% have some type of sleep-related disorder that can cause fragmentation of sleep (Mellinger *et al.*, 1985).

Sleep deprivation has many consequences, including poor educational or occupational performance, an increased risk of developing physical and psychiatric disorders and increased overall morbidity (Ford and Kamerow, 1989).

The downside of inadequate sleep is the impairment of daytime functioning that it causes. Feeling drowsy whilst driving a motor vehicle or operating machinery can have dangerous if not catastrophic consequences. It can also adversely influence the decision-making process.

Sleepiness has been directly linked to road traffic accidents. Serious accidents have been shown to peak between 01.00 and 04.00, the time when

people are normally asleep, and 13.00 and 16.00, when people are biologi-
cally at a low point. Some the world's biggest catastrophes have also been
attributed to the people responsible being sleep deprived (Mitler *et al.*, 1988).

The economic cost of daytime drowsiness is enormous. Sleep deprivation
therefore constitutes a major public health concern.

CLASSIFICATION OF SLEEP DISORDERS

The International Classification of Sleep Disorders (ICSD, 1990) is divided
into three broad categories: primary sleep disorders; sleep disorders due to
medical or psychiatric conditions; and 'proposed sleep disorders'. The last
category is made up of a group of conditions which it is thought require
further study before they can be regarded as discrete, diagnosable conditions
(e.g. menstrual-associated sleep disorder, sleep-related laryngospasm, sleep
choking syndrome). Primary sleep disorders are further subdivided into
dyssomnias and parasomnias.

Dyssomnias are disorders that cause either difficulty in initiating and/or
maintaining sleep or excessive sleepiness (hypersomnia). They may be intrinsic or extrinsic.

The intrinsic sleep disorders include those that primarily cause insomnia
(such as psychophysiological insomnia, idiopathic insomnia or sleep state
misperception), those that cause both insomnia and hypersomnia (e.g. the
sleep apnoea syndrome) and those that cause hypersomnia (e.g. narcolepsy).

Similarly, extrinsic sleep disorders may lead to insomnia (e.g. adjustment
sleep disorder, inadequate sleep hygiene, environmental sleep disorder,
altitude insomnia and limit-setting sleep disorder), insomnia and hypersomnia (e.g. alcohol-dependent sleep disorder, stimulant-dependent sleep disorder) or hypersomnia (e.g. insufficient sleep syndrome).

Also included in the dyssomnias are circadian rhythm sleep disorders. In
these conditions there is disturbance of the biological clock and included in
the category are conditions such as jet lag syndrome, shift work sleep disorder, and delayed and advanced sleep phase syndromes.

Parasomnias are unusual events, which occur at various stages of sleep.
Some are arousal disorders (e.g. sleepwalking, sleep terrors), some are associated with sleep–wake transition (e.g. sleep talking) and some with REM sleep
(e.g. nightmares, sleep paralysis), whilst others have no particular association
(e.g. enuresis, bruxism and sleep-related abnormal swallowing syndrome).

Sleep disturbance may be associated with a variety of psychiatric disorders
(e.g. mood disorders, anxiety disorders, psychoses and panic disorder), and
with neurological conditions (e.g. dementia and parkinsonism). Sleep can
also be disturbed in some medical conditions (e.g. gastro-oesophageal reflux
and nocturnal asthma).

Altogether the ICSD lists some 84 distinct sleep disorders. Of these 84 disorders, the 10 commonest are:

- adjustment sleep disorder
- psychophysiological insomnia
- inadequate sleep hygiene
- mood disorder
- obstructive sleep apnoea
- circadian rhythm disorder
- shift work sleep disorder
- alcohol dependent sleep disorder
- periodic limb movements
- fibrositis syndrome.

Of particular importance to primary care are the concepts of psychophysiological insomnia, idiopathic insomnia and sleep state misperception. Psychophysiological insomnia is defined as 'a disorder of somatized tension and learned sleep-preventing associations that results in a complaint of insomnia and associated decreased functioning during wakefulness'.

Idiopathic insomnia is 'a lifelong inability to obtain adequate sleep that is presumably due to an abnormality of the neurological control of the sleep–wake system'.

Sleep state misperception is 'a disorder in which a complaint of insomnia or excessive sleepiness occurs without objective evidence of sleep disturbance'.

DSM-IV (*Diagnostic and Statistical Manual of Mental Disorders*, fourth edition; American Psychiatric Association, 1994) adopts a somewhat simpler approach to the classification of sleep disorders as does ICD-10 (International Classification of Diseases, 10th revision; WHO, 1992). DSM-IV is divided into primary sleep disorders, sleep disorders related to another mental disorder and other sleep disorders.

Primary sleep disorders are further divided into the dyssomnias (primary insomnia, primary hypersomnia, narcolepsy, breathing-related sleep disorder, circadian rhythm sleep disorder and dyssomnia not otherwise specified) and parasomnias (sleep terror disorder, sleepwalking disorder and parasomnia not otherwise specified). Sleep disorders related to another mental disorder includes those insomnias associated with Axis I or Axis II disorders, whilst included in the category 'other sleep disorders' are sleep disorders caused by general medical conditions and those that are substance-induced.

The criteria for primary insomnia are: 'a predominant complaint of difficulty initiating or maintaining sleep; or non-restorative sleep, for at least 1 month'; it should cause clinically significant distress or impairment in social, occupational or other areas of functioning; should not occur exclusively during the course of another sleep disorder, nor during the course of another mental disorder; and should not be due to the direct physiological effects of a substance or a general medical condition.

ICD-10 separates 'non-organic' sleep disorders (F51) from those considered organic such as the Kleine–Levin syndrome and those considered non-psychogenic such as narcolepsy and cataplexy, disorders of the sleep–wake schedule, sleep apnoea, episodic movement disorders and enuresis. The category 'non-organic sleep disorders' is divided into dyssomnias (non-organic insomnia, non-organic hypersomnia and non-organic disorder of the sleep–wake schedule) and parasomnias (sleepwalking, sleep terrors and nightmares).

The diagnostic guidelines for non-organic insomnia require the following 'essential clinical features for a definite diagnosis':

1. The complaint is either of difficulty falling asleep or maintaining sleep or of poor quality of sleep.
2. The sleep disturbance has occurred at least three times a week for at least 1 month.
3. There is a preoccupation with the sleeplessness and excessive concern over its consequences at night and during the day.
4. The unsatisfactory quantity and/or quality of sleep either causes marked distress or interferes with social and occupational functioning.

A simple and very practical alternative to the rather complex classifications so far outlined, and especially useful when considering insomnias, is to use the '5 Ps', i.e. could the cause be physical, physiological, psychological, psychiatric or pharmacological?

Physical causes include pain of any kind, paroxysmal nocturnal dyspnoea, asthma, gastro-oesophageal reflux, tinnitus and prostatism. Physiological causes include unsuitable sleeping environment, late night eating, late night exercise and other deficiencies in sleep hygiene, jet lag and changes in shift working practices. Stress, tension, grief and undue concern about sleeping would fall into the psychological category. Many psychiatric disorders (anxiety, depression, mania and dementia for example) are associated with poor or disturbed sleep. Finally, insomnia may be pharmacologically induced either by prescribed medication – beta-adrenergic blockers, steroids, stimulants and some antidepressants – or by social 'drugs' such as alcohol, caffeine and nicotine.

Systematic use of the '5 P' approach should lead to the identification of the majority of sleep disorders.

DIAGNOSIS

When addressing a complaint of poor, inadequate, disturbed or unsatisfactory sleep, appropriate management will depend upon making a diagnosis. Most insomnias have a predisposing cause and the diagnosis of primary or non-organic insomnia should only be made by exclusion. The importance of a comprehensive sleep history cannot be over-stressed.

Questions to be explored in a 'sleep history' include:

- How long have you had difficulty sleeping?
- What was your sleep pattern before you had a problem?
- How long does it take you to fall asleep?
- For how long do you sleep?
- Is the problem falling asleep, staying asleep, waking early, or a combination of these?
- Have there been other times in your life when you have had similar problems?
- Do you consider the duration of your sleep adequate?
- Do you consider your sleep satisfactory?
- Do you wake feeling refreshed?
- Are you tired and sleepy during the day?
- Do you snore?
- Does your bed partner complain about your snoring or restlessness?
- What do you expect of sleep?
- For how long do you think you should sleep?
- Is your sleep disturbed by repetitive movements or restless legs?

This history taking should go on to explore any concomitant physical disorders, enquire about any prescribed medication being taken, and about the use of caffeine, alcohol, nicotine and any recreational drugs. Enquiry needs to be made about any current stress or concerns, and an assessment of mood state (depressed, anxious) is vitally important. Information is also required about the sleeping environment, sleep–wake timetabling, evening habits (eating, exercising, use of the bedroom), occupational and work schedules, response to treatment already tried (alcohol, over-the-counter preparations, prescribed preparations), and any family history of sleep problems.

In some circumstances it may be helpful to interview the bed partner. He or she might be able to provide valuable additional information about the patient's sleep pattern, nocturnal movements, snoring, apnoeic episodes and so on. It may also be helpful to encourage the patient to keep a sleep diary, although he or she should be warned not to be too obsessional about it. The information obtained may be very subjective. Nevertheless, it can give some indication of the overall sleep pattern as well as providing a baseline against which subsequent improvement can be measured. Keeping a diary may also assist patients in gaining some insight into their sleep difficulties.

Sleep apnoea

Special reference needs to be made to obstructive sleep apnoea. Patients who have this condition may principally complain of tiredness during the day, attribute it to poor quality sleep at night, and may even request the prescription of a hypnotic agent to resolve the problem. Sleep apnoea is associated with persistent crescendo-like snoring. Each apnoeic episode leads to a microarousal and because such arousals may occur hundreds of times during the night the accumulated sleep deficit can lead to substantial daytime drowsiness. Risk factors for obstructive sleep apnoea include obesity and excessive alcohol consumption. A useful indicator of the likelihood of sleep apnoea occurring is collar size. Sleep apnoeics usually have a fat neck with a collar size of 17 or more. The risk of sleep apnoea occurring increases with age and it is associated with a higher than normal risk of cardiovascular abnormalities and sudden death. There is a close association between sleep apnoea and accidents on the road and at work.

The hallmark of obstructive sleep apnoea is daytime drowsiness. Unless a careful history is taken (often including an interview with the bed partner) there is a danger that this may be attributed to simple insomnia and hypnotic agents will be prescribed. These will only exacerbate the problem and are contraindicated. Treatment of sleep apnoea includes reduction in alcohol intake, weight loss, changing sleeping positions and in severe cases continuous positive airways pressure (CPAP) or even pharyngeal surgery.

Parasomnias and narcolepsy

This chapter has been principally concerned with the dyssomnias (especially insomnia) and their causes and management. With the exception of nocturnal enuresis, the majority of parasomnias will need specialist referral from primary care. This will also invariably be so in cases of narcolepsy.

MANAGEMENT OF INSOMNIA

Education and information

In managing insomnia an initial explanation of the nature of sleep is required (World Psychiatric Association, 1992). An imponderable is how much sleep an individual requires. Although the average person requires between 7 and 8 hours nightly, some individuals are short sleepers, whereas others are long. Daytime function and drowsiness are probably the best indicators of adequacy; individuals require sufficient sleep to keep them alert and free from drowsiness during the day.

A brief explanation of the normal architecture of sleep will be helpful, indicating that the deepest sleep occurs during the first few hours of the night. Thereafter sleep is shallower and punctuated by periods when dreaming may occur and also by arousals, which may vary in duration from being so short that they are not remembered or longer periods of wakefulness. With increasing age, sleep requirement tends to diminish and is associated with longer periods of being awake in bed at night. It is important to emphasize that this 'fragmentation' is normal and natural. It should give no cause for concern and usually the individual will fall asleep again after a period of wakefulness. Age-related changes in sleep pattern may conflict with an individual's 'expectation' of sleep. Many people feel that they need 'a good 8 hours' of sleep at night and may even demand a hypnotic unnecessarily if they do not get it.

Elderly people tend to sleep or 'nap' during the day. They should appreciate that this may well reduce their nocturnal sleep requirement. Children require longer periods of uninterrupted sleep than adults. Problems usually arise through inadequate limit setting. Adolescents may have too short or displaced (i.e. up all night, asleep all day) sleep cycles.

Sleep hygiene

Before any other type of treatment is envisaged, attention should be paid to what is now known as sleep hygiene. This essentially means emphasizing practices or habits that encourage sleep, eliminating or reducing those that interfere with it, and attempting to reinforce the natural rhythm of sleeping and waking. The basic principles of good sleep hygiene are:

1. *Sleep environment.* A proper sleep environment is required: dark and quiet, not too hot or too cold, not too humid, and in a bed that is both comfortable and in good condition (i.e. not likely to cause physical problems that disturb sleep).

2. *Avoidance of substances or activities that may disturb sleep.* Caffeine (contained in tea, coffee, cocoa, cola drinks and other beverages) should be avoided in the late evening by insomniacs. It can be arousing and consequently disturb sleep. Caffeine sensitivity increases with age. Nicotine can disturb sleep and late evening smoking should be discouraged.

Caution needs to be exercised in the consumption of alcohol, especially if this is excessive. Whereas alcohol may induce sleep, it can, by virtue of its short half-life and consequent withdrawal effects, lead to arousal and consequent fragmentation of sleep. Small amounts of alcohol may be permissible, but large amounts are certainly contraindicated.

Vigorous exercise during the day may be conducive to sound sleep, but if taken too close to the retiring time, is likely to be disruptive. Exercise taken in the evening should be gentle.

Eating large meals late in the day will also cause sleep disturbance.

3. *Reinforcing the natural rhythm of alertness during the day and sleepiness at night.* One of the problems that insomniacs often have is their chaotic timetabling. Opinions vary somewhat on the question of timetabling. It could

be argued that keeping regular hours is important, i.e. going to bed at the same time each evening and getting up at the same time each morning (avoiding 'lying in' at weekends and on holidays). Alternatively, patients should be advised not to go to bed until they feel sleepy. However, what does seem to be important is rising at the same time every morning as this influences the setting of the biological clock.

4. *Setting the mood for sleep.* Entering the bedroom should be the 'cue' for going to sleep. Bedrooms are for sleeping in and not places in which to eat, work, watch television and so on. Reinforcement can be provided by a regular bedtime routine.

5. *Avoid sleeping during the day.* Whereas some people might find a short 'nap' during the day helpful (e.g. when feeling sleepy after a long period of motorway driving), prolonged napping during the day will provide some of the total sleep requirement and lead to disturbed sleep at night.

6. *Don't take your worries to bed.* Individuals preoccupied with worries or anxieties should try, if possible, to resolve them before going to bed or endeavour to leave them until the next day. Some may benefit from being taught relaxation or distraction techniques.

Pharmacotherapy

If education, reassurance and attention to sleep hygiene are ineffective, it may be necessary to have recourse to pharmacotherapeutic agents. Historically, many agents have been used as hypnotic agents. The perfect hypnotic would have the following profile:

1. It should induce sleep rapidly.
2. It should maintain sleep adequately.
3. It should allow the taker to wake refreshed and without a hangover.
4. It should not disturb the normal architecture of sleep.
5. It should not cause rebound insomnia, withdrawal effects or dependence.
6. It should be safe if consumed in overdose.
7. It should not cause sedation or behavioural toxicity during the following day.
8. It should not cause any interference in cognitive function or memory.
9. It should not have active metabolites that have different characteristics to those of the parent compound.

Unfortunately no such hypnotic exists. Nevertheless, these criteria should be used to assess the features of any particular agent. Agents previously used or currently available include:

1. *Alcohol and opium*. Historically these are the oldest hypnotic agents. Clearly their use is contraindicated.

2. *Chloral derivatives*. These are amongst the oldest of the currently available hypnotic agents. They have a number of disadvantages: they may cause high dose-dependence, gastric irritation and skin rashes, and may be dangerous in overdose.

3. *Barbiturates*. For many years these were the most widely used hypnotic agents. However, their side-effect profile has made them obsolete, i.e. daytime sedation, dependence, toxicity in overdose, and induction of liver enzymes.

4. *Chlormethiazole*. The principal problem with this compound is its high propensity to cause dependence. It can cause gastric irritation and skin rashes and is not safe when taken in overdose.

5. *Antihistamines*. Although antihistamines have been and still are widely used, they have a number of disadvantages: many have long half-lives and cause daytime drowsiness, they can produce anticholinergic side effects and are toxic in overdose. Whether they restore normal sleep or are just 'sedative' is debatable.

6. *Antidepressants*. Sedative antidepressants have been widely used in low doses to treat insomnia. However, many, particularly tricyclic antidepressants, disrupt normal sleep architecture. The older antidepressants should only be used when there is clear evidence of a primary psychiatric disorder (e.g. major depressive disorder with associated sleep disturbance).

7. *Herbal products*. Traditionally, a number of herbal products have been used to induce sleep. They include *Anemone pulsatilla*, camomile, valerian and verbena. Evidence for efficacy from controlled clinical trials is lacking.

8. *Hot milky drinks*. Another tradition suggests that taking a hot milky drink at bedtime induces sleep. The effect may be due to the fact that milk contains tryptophan, a precursor of serotonin.

9. *Benzodiazepines and allied compounds (cyclopyrrolones and imidazopyridines)* Table 1. Benzodiazepines, and compounds such as the cyclopyrrolones and imidazopyridines, which although chemically unrelated, have a similar pharmacological action (i.e. are ligands of the gamma-aminobutyric acid (GABA)/benzodiazepine molecular complex) are the most appropriate and most widely used hypnotic agents. Collectively these compounds have

Table 1. Characteristics of selected benzodiazepines.

	Flurazepam	Nitrazepam	Temazepam	Triazolam	Zopiclone	Zolpidem
Active metabolite	Yes	No	No	No	Yes	Yes
Peak plasma concentration (h)	30–40 min	2	1.25	2	0.5–1.5	2.2
Rate of elimination	Slow	Slow	Intermediate	Rapid	Rapid	Rapid
Elimination half-life (h)	47–100	30	9.5–12.4	1.5–5.5	3.5–6	1.5–2.4
	(long)	(long)	(intermediate)	(short)	(short)	(short)

been referred to as benzodiazepine receptor agonists. Traditionally, hypnotics have been classified according to their elimination half-lives, i.e. the time taken for the concentration in blood to fall by 50%. Obviously, the hypnotic effect depends upon dose, presuming that there is a threshold at which a hypnotic effect is achieved, and of the rate of absorption. Metabolism may also be important because a metabolite, if produced, may have a longer half-life than the parent compound. Nevertheless, elimination half-life has proved to be a useful indicator of profile. Thus, benzodiazepines and allied agents can be classified as long-, medium- and short-acting.

Long-acting compounds include flurazepam, nitrazepam and fluni-trazepam. Because of their long half-lives these compounds are likely to exert effects beyond the duration of normal sleep, leading to daytime sedation and possible behavioural toxicity. They are also likely to accumulate when regular nightly doses are used. Half-life duration may depend upon other factors, particularly, for example, age, and consequently the likelihood and damage of accumulation may be greater in elderly subjects.

Intermediate-acting compounds include temazepam and lormetazepam. Triazolam, midazolam, zopiclone (a cyclopyrrolone) and zolpidem (an imida-zopyridine) are all short-acting. By virtue of their somewhat different binding characteristics at the GABA/benzodiazepine molecular complex it has been postulated that the cyclopyrrolone and imidazopyridine hypnotics are less likely to cause rebound and dependence. All benzodiazepines and allied hypnotics, with the exception of zolpidem, affect sleep architecture. Choice of compound will depend on the type of sleep disorder and its characteristics, and whether the objective is to induce sleep, maintain it, or both. Preservation of daytime alertness is of vital importance and only in exceptional circumstances is the use of compounds with a long half-life not contraindicated.

USING HYPNOTICS

A National Institutes of Mental Health Consensus Development Conference on Drugs and Insomnia (National Institute of Mental Health, 1984) suggested that 'sleep promoting drug therapy should be considered for patients when they are significantly troubled by the presence of inadequate sleep, or when the physician is concerned about the deleterious impact of disturbed sleep on the patient's health, safety and well-being'. The conference suggested three major categories of insomnia based on duration: transient, short-term and long-term.

Transient insomnia is defined as 'a normal sleeper who experiences an acute stress or stressful situation lasting less than a week (e.g. hospitalization) or a disruption of the biological sleep-regulating mechanism by a change in schedules due to air travel over time zones or a recent work-schedule change'.

Short-term insomnia usually 'is associated with longer situational stress (e.g. grief, often related to work and family life or serious medical illness)'. The term is used when insomnia lasts from 1 to 3 weeks.

Long-term insomnia has a duration of more than a month. Although it can occur *per se* (i.e. psychopathological insomnia and that due to inadequate sleep hygiene), it is frequently associated with underlying conditions (e.g. anxiety, depression, obstructive sleep apnoea, medication or alcohol induced, periodic limb movements etc.). Hypnotics, preferably those with shorter duration of action, are entirely appropriate for treating transient and short-term insomnia. Caution is needed, however, to avoid impairment of compensatory and coping reactions to stress. In short-term insomnia, vigilance is required to avoid an insidious slide into long-term use. Intermittent use may be helpful.

Long-term insomnia is more difficult to treat. If an underlying disorder has been identified (e.g. depression or a painful condition) this should be treated first. A short initial course of hypnotics may be justified until control of the underlying disorder is achieved.

Treatment of the long-term or life-long poor sleeper is especially difficult. Intermittent hypnotic use may be appropriate in some circumstances. Treatment should commence with the lowest recommended dose and only be increased if this proves to be ineffective. Tapering is recommended when withdrawing high doses. Care needs to be exercised in elderly patients because age-related changes in metabolism and kinetics may lead to accumulation. Unsupervised repeat prescriptions should not be permitted in any circumstances.

Patients should be made aware that discontinuation of hypnotic therapy, even after short courses, may result in some rebound insomnia.

Following treatment of long-term insomnia or when discontinuing hypnotic therapy in long-term users, abrupt discontinuation should be avoided and a tapered withdrawal regime instituted. Unless this practice is observed, and even sometimes when it is, withdrawal effects may be experienced. Withdrawal effects include anxiety, loss of appetite and weight, vertigo, palpitations, sweating, tremor and sometimes perceptual distortions such as hyperacusis, photophobia, paraesthesia and hypersensitivity to touch and pain.

REFERENCES

American Psychiatric Association (1994). *Diagnostic Criteria from DSM-IV.* American Psychiatric Association, Washington, DC.

Ford, D.E. and Kamerow, D.B. (1989). Epidemiological study of sleep disturbances and psychiatric disorders. *JAMA* **262**, 1479–1524.

ICSD (1990). Diagnostic Classification Steering Committee: Thorpy, M.J., Chairman. *International Classification of Sleep Disorders: Diagnostic and Coding Manual.* American Sleep Disorders Association, Rochester, MN.

Mellinger, G.D., Balter, M.B. and Uhlenhuth, E.H. (1985). Insomnia and 'its treatment'. *Arch Gen Psychiatry* **42**, 225–232.

Mitler, M.M., Carskadon, M.A., Czeisler, J. *et al.* (1988). Catastrophes, sleep and public policy: consensus report. *Sleep* **11**, 100–109.

Mniszek, D.H. (1988). Brighton sleep survey: a study of sleep in 20 to 45 years olds. *Int Med Res* **16**, 61–65.

NIMH (1984). Drugs and insomnia. National Institutes of Mental Health Consensus Development Conference. **251**, 2410–2414.

World Health Organization (1992). *The ICD-10 Classification of Mental and Behavioural Disorders. Clinical Descriptions and Diagnostic Guidelines.* WHO, Geneva.

World Psychiatric Association Presidential Educational Programme (1992). *The Management of Insomnia: Guidelines for Clinical Practice.* The Upjohn Company. Pragmaton.

Benzodiazepines
Edited by Michael R. Trimble and Ian Hindmarch
© 2000 Wrightson Biomedical Publishing Ltd

4

The Use of Benzodiazepines in the Management of Anxiety: A Clinical Perspective

D.D.R. WILLIAMS and J. SMITH

Cefn Coed Hospital, Swansea, Wales UK

INTRODUCTION

Anxiety is a universal human emotion occurring readily in response to threat or stress. Its development is easy to understand and it has a protective energizing benefit. Unfortunately it can occur in inappropriate circumstances and to a degree that is distressing, disabling and sometimes paralysing. As anxiety and its associated features appear so frequently, every health professional should have a good and easy grasp of its symptoms and signs. As the emphasis in this chapter is on its management only, a reminder of the key symptoms of anxiety follow.

Anxiety is the most common form of mental illness and there are two groups of symptoms: psychological and physical. The hallmark of the disorder is an overwhelming feeling of fear, dread and apprehension, a feeling of tension, of suspense and the foreboding that something terrible is going to happen. Linked with this awful apprehension and being keyed up is the secondary problem of inability to sleep. Insomnia is an integral component of anxiety and it occurs even when there is severe physical exhaustion. The psychological symptoms are linked with a number of physical symptoms, which are due to overactivity of the sympathetic nervous system. These include: dry mouth, butterflies in the upper abdomen, palpitations, tightness of the throat, throbbing and tension headaches, loose motions and urinary frequency.

Anxiety can be entirely due to psychological mechanisms. In addition, it is frequently found in association with physical disease, particularly illness that is serious and life-threatening. As anxiety is such a common disorder and its presentation so varied it is vital for every health professional to be able to recognize it easily and to feel confident in giving sound advice about its management. In clinical practice, it is important to be able to distinguish symptoms of anxiety that are not associated with other psychiatric symptoms such as depression, motor restlessness or psychotic phenomena. When anxiety is only a part of a bigger psychiatric problem, the benzodiazepines have only a small part to play. The major thrust of management then is directed towards the more severe symptoms and is likely to include the use of antidepressant and neuroleptic drugs.

The clinical states of anxiety in which the benzodiazepines have an important part to play have been identified by the time-honoured diagnostic concepts of anxiety neurosis, anxiety reaction, phobic disorders and anxiety states. These terms are still used extensively in clinical practice but are being replaced by the terminology of the ICD-10 (International Classification of Diseases, 10th revision; World Health Organization, 1992) and DSM-IV (*Diagnostic and Statistical Manual of Mental Disorders*, fourth edition; American Psychiatric Association, 1994) manuals. The majority of patients seen in clinical practice with uncomplicated symptoms of anxiety are included within the diagnostic categories of general anxiety disorder, panic and phobic disorders.

General anxiety disorder can usually be understood in terms of the individual's personality make-up, predicament, life stresses and problems. Even when the symptoms are quite severe they can be eased considerably by a warm, empathic and supportive interview, but the improvement is short-lived. In order to obtain a sustained improvement the use of medication for symptom control must be considered.

HISTORICAL BACKGROUND

In order to understand the current use and role of drugs in the management of anxiety it is necessary to have an understanding of the history of the problem so that the contemporary scene can be evaluated from the perspective of what has happened over the centuries, and particularly over the recent past. Without this knowledge the real thrust of current developments and the continuing role of the benzodiazepines in the management of anxiety disorders cannot be adequately judged.

Alcohol and opium have been used for thousands of years to relieve anxiety. It is impossible to place a date on the time when carbohydrates were first fermented to produce alcoholic beverages. The process was well known to the Greeks and Romans and probably to still more remote times. The science of distillation was introduced to Western Europe by the Arabs

(Lader, 1991) in the Middle Ages. Brandy was described as *aqua vitae* (water of life) and considered to be a panacea. Whisky was regarded in the same way and the word is derived from the Gaelic *uisgebetha: uisge* – water and *betha* – life (later contracted to *usquebaugh*). In the eighteenth century cheap spirits in the form of gin became available and soon the dangers of its extensive consumption became apparent.

Opium was widely used in Britain during the nineteenth and early twentieth century mainly in the form of laudanum, a tincture of opium. Again it was considered to be a panacea for a wide range of disorders. Berridge (1999) gives a scholarly account of its use and drug control policy. Acceptance of opium was so general that horticultural societies gave awards for growing the poppy and medical practitioners were amongst the prizewinners. Berridge outlines how, as the pharmaceutical and medical professions gained power, they redefined opium use as a cause of concern and regular use as 'a disease'. Plant (1999) considers this book as essential reading for anyone interested in the relationship between humanity and psychoactive drugs.

Lader (1991) has provided a summary of new psychotropic sedative drugs that were introduced in the middle of the nineteenth century, starting with potassium bromide. By the latter part of the eighteenth century bromides were widely used but eventually their dependence potential was realized. Around the same time, synthesized organic preparations became available. The first two were chloral hydrate and paraldehyde. These were also associated with abuse and dependence. Paraldehyde has been obsolete for some time but chloral hydrate still has limited use as a hypnotic in the elderly.

Barbituric acid was synthesized by Adolf von Bayer and the first hypnotic barbiturate, barbital or Veronal, was introduced in 1903. This was followed by numerous other products, 50 of which were marketed. Other compounds with similar pharmacological properties were introduced but had to be discarded because their dependence potential and toxicity became apparent. Slater and Roth (1969) provide a picture of the extent that the bromides and barbiturates were prescribed in the early and mid-twentieth century. Before the Second World War, 40% of the medicines prescribed to panel patients in Britain contained bromides; but by the 1960s their use had been diminished and was replaced by barbiturates. In 1957–59, barbiturates constituted between 19% and 20% of the total number of prescriptions for drugs of all kinds during those years. In the post-war period, the barbiturate drugs were regarded as very important in the management of anxiety and sleeplessness despite the recognition of the two principal dangers: suicide and addiction. In 1950, meprobamate 'Miltown' or 'Equanil' was developed and promoted as an anxiolytic, but by 1964 its dangers of causing physical dependence had been realized and it was replaced by the benzodiazepines.

INTRODUCTION OF THE BENZODIAZEPINES

The benzodiazepines were first synthesized in the 1930s and in 1960 chlor-diazepoxide was introduced followed by its even more successful relative diazepam in 1963. There is no doubt that the usage of benzodiazepines quickly escalated. In some circles this was seen as a new development; however, what was happening was that the benzodiazepines were replacing the barbiturates in the management of anxiety and insomnia. Naturally the main reason for this change was the much improved safety profile of the benzodiazepines.

The prescriptions for benzodiazepines continued to increase, reaching a peak in the mid-1970s. The situation in Wales is set out in Table 1 and there are no reasons to believe that the pattern of prescribing is any different to the remainder of the UK.

Table 1. *Benzodiazepines in Wales, UK. Number of prescriptions.*

Drug group	1979	1985	1988	1989	1990	1997
Temazepam	59.9	420.8	573.9	578.1	571.4	532.4
Nitrazepam	684.1	413.1	323.9	328.6	310.6	232.6
Diazepam	680.0	404.5	343.3	331.3	321.0	469.6
Lorazepam	126.8	230.9	138.1	138.4	125.2	75.4
Chlordiazepoxide (incl. hydrochloride)	118.3	78.9	61.4	59.3	55.4	37.0
Total	1669.1	1548.2	1440.6	1435.7	1383.6	1347.0

All data in 000s.

It can be seen that following the peak in the 1970s there has been a steady decline over the next 20 years in the numbers of scripts dispensed. In the last 10 years, there has been a shift away from prescribing anxiolytic drugs with short half-lives (e.g. lorazepam) in favour of those with longer half-lives (e.g. diazepam). This is based on the rationale that a discontinuation syndrome is less likely to occur when withholding a benzodiazepine with a long half-life.

The figures for hypnotic prescriptions show a marked shift in the early 1980s with temazepam being substituted for nitrazepam in many instances. Since then the nitrazepam prescriptions have gradually declined while those for temazepam rose until the late 1980s. The decline in hypnotic prescription by 1997 might be explained by the availability of alternative hypnotics such as zopiclone and zolpidem. The requirement that possession of temazepam needed to be accompanied by proof of prescription may also have dissuaded some clinicians from dispensing this medication.

The extensive use of the benzodiazepines during the 1970s and early 1980s was beginning to raise doubts in a few clinicians' minds. It was noted that a large cohort of long-term users was becoming established. Worries began to emerge that patients on therapeutic doses were becoming physically dependant but, as this was at variance with accepted teachings on dependence, the idea was dismissed. Eventually, research findings showed it to be the case but controversy raged over whether it was a common feature.

COMMITTEE ON SAFETY OF MEDICINE GUIDELINES

These anxieties led in turn to the UK Committee on Safety of Medicines (1988) and the Royal College of Psychiatrists (1988) issuing very stringent guidelines about the use of benzodiazepine drugs. The Committee on Safety of Medicines recommended that the use of benzodiazepines should be limited in the following ways.

Uses

As anxiolytics:

1. Benzodiazepines are indicated for the short-term relief (2–4 weeks only) of anxiety that is severe, disabling or subjecting the individual to unacceptable distress, occurring alone or in association with insomnia or short-term psychosomatic, organic or psychotic illness.
2. The use of benzodiazepines to treat short-term 'mild' anxiety is inappropriate and unsuitable.

As hypnotics:

3. Benzodiazepines should be used to treat insomnia only when it is severe, disabling or subjecting the individual to extreme distress.

Dose

1. The lowest dose that can control the symptoms should be used. It should not be continued beyond 4 weeks.
2. Long-term chronic use is not recommended.
3. Treatment should always be reduced gradually.
4. Patients who have taken benzodiazepines for a long time may require a longer period during which doses are reduced.
5. When a benzodiazepine is used as a hypnotic, treatment should, preferably, be intermittent.

Precautions

1. Benzodiazepines should not be used alone to treat depression or anxiety associated with depression. Suicide may be precipitated in such patients.

2. They should not be used for phobic or obsessional states.
3. They should not be used for the treatment of chronic psychosis.
4. In cases of loss or bereavement, psychological adjustment may be inhibited by benzodiazepines.
5. Disinhibiting effects may be manifested in various ways. Benzodiazepines may precipitate suicide in patients who are depressed, and aggressive behaviour towards self and others. Extreme caution should therefore be used when prescribing benzodiazepines for patients with personality disorders.

THE EFFECT OF THE GUIDELINES

At the time when the guidelines were published there were vociferous critics (Williams, 1988). It was felt that the guidelines were an inhibiting and constraining influence on good psychiatric practice and that there was a danger that this group of drugs would be banned, creating a serious gap in the armamentarium of effective treatment for anxiety and insomnia. To a clinician it appeared that the guidelines had been prepared mainly by psychiatrists with a major commitment to academic work and with a bias towards undertaking trials with new drugs. The question of whether such a body of opinion was ideally placed to form guidelines about the use of benzodiazepines in contemporary routine medical and psychiatric practice was posed.

There is little doubt that the guidelines made a considerable impact on the number of prescriptions that were given and also altered the attitude of many doctors towards this group of drugs. In addition to a reduction in the number of benzodiazepine prescriptions that were prescribed, it is necessary to consider what other consequences the guidelines have produced.

1. Some family doctors and some psychiatrists took the moral highground and saw it as their responsibility to rapidly wean patients off the benzodiazepines and to stop using them completely. Some behaved as apparatchiks, zealously implementing government policy. Tensions developed between psychiatrists and primary care doctors when the two parties had differing views about this issue. On occasions family doctors would not prescribe benzodiazepines even when recommend by a specialist. Many primary and secondary care doctors, possibly the silent majority, continued to prescribe these drugs but frequently felt unsupported and working at variance with government policy.

2. Soon a new trend in prescribing was emerging and many had reservations about it. This was the use of a whole range of other drugs to treat

anxiety and insomnia: drugs that were less suitable and had far more trouble-some side effects than the benzodiazepines. Low dose phenothiazines, beta-blockers, tricyclic antidepressants, antihistamines and latterly the serotonin-selective reuptake inhibitor (SSRI) drugs were being used to treat uncomplicated anxiety disorders.

3. There is another serious criticism of this development in addition to the fact that these alternative drugs are less suitable than the benzodiazepines for treating anxiety and insomnia. Psychiatry is not a discipline in which it is easy to learn and acquire the basic rudiments. Particularly with such a plethora of psychotropic drugs, psychiatrists and consultant psychiatrists in particular have a responsibility to be seen to be promoting and to comply themselves with the basic ground rules for the prescribing of psychotropic medication. Essentially there are three groups of psychoactive drugs: the anxiolytics and hypnotics; antidepressants; and, thirdly, the neuroleptics or major tranquillizers. In order to promote good practice, these drugs should only be prescribed for the particular condition for which they are indicated. The vast majority of psychotropic drugs are prescribed by family doctors and it is very important for them to see clearly and to be reminded about the broad pattern of prescribing that psychiatrists adopt and use. This new trend of prescribing almost any drug with sedative qualities for anxiety and insom-nia undermines these important ground rules and degrades good psychiatric practice.

4. In general hospitals, it was common to see patients being rapidly weaned off benzodiazepines, the view being that every patient on these drugs must be weaned off them and that the benzodiazepines must never be prescribed for them again. Frequently this was done far too quickly and anecdotally elderly patients were reported to have never recovered completely from being destabilized in this way.

5. In parallel with these developments, there were sensational programmes on television highlighting the dangers of benzodiazepines and many of them caused considerable distress to patients who relied on these drugs for their well-being. After each one it was not uncommon to see a patient who had stopped his or her medication suddenly and had become very distressed. After being bombarded by the media patients had to be constantly reassured that taking psychoactive drugs was a clinical necessity and essential for their continuing well-being.

6. Following the release of the guidelines it became clear that there were many patients with persistent anxiety and severe intractable insomnia who were being denied effective treatment. When working in the local prison it

was very common to find prisoners suffering from severe generalized anxiety and insomnia. Some were anxious men enduring their first term of imprisonment and their suffering was easy to see from the extent they had bitten their nails. Their fingers were like red inflamed drumsticks. Naturally it was not always easy to decide who should receive treatment particularly as the ethos of the prison was to view these reactions as part and parcel of what being in prison entailed. Despite this culture, it was felt that the humanitarian and ethical approach was that the inmates who developed severe symptoms should receive proper and adequate treatment.

A CONTEMPORARY REVIEW OF THE GUIDELINES

Eleven years have passed since the guidelines were published and it is timely to take stock of the position and to re-examine the recommendations that were made. At the time of their publication many doctors considered them to be very harsh and that is still the view. It is worthwhile focusing on some of the main issues.

1. Consider the recommendation about hypnotics: 'Benzodiazepines should be used to treat insomnia only when it is severe, disabling or subjecting the individual to extreme distress. The lowest dose which can control the symptoms should be used. It should not be continued beyond four weeks.' It is not unreasonable to suggest that the committee members who prepared the guidelines had not suffered from insomnia themselves and the impression is given that they had not dealt in a sensitive and helpful way with patients with sleep problems. In psychiatric practice, insomnia is due to either a mental illness or severe personal problems and these difficulties are not going to be resolved in 4 weeks. Since the guidelines were produced, the impression is received that many doctors are more preoccupied with not prescribing hypnotics than with acknowledging the importance of sleep and the need to treat insomnia effectively. Sleep is essential for well-being; it plays an important part in the healing process, and in recovery and recuperation. In contemporary medical culture, it is often necessary to spell this out. Greater emphasis needs to be placed on the importance of high-quality sleep (Oswald, 1986).

2. Since the guidelines were published, doctors are being increasingly asked to review their prescribing pattern in the light of evidence-based clinical guidelines which are derived particularly from information drawn from all available primary sources but particularly from random-allocation clinical trials. Clinicians are very conscious that the evidence-based medicine

approach must be balanced and modulated by experiential perspectives. The results from double blind trials must be considered in the light of insights gained from treating individual patients. This vignette from the Personal View column of the *British Medical Journal* demonstrates the importance of the experiential perspective (Khursandi, 1998).

This is a moving account by a young anaesthetist about her depressive illness. She starts by describing how her mother committed suicide by hanging when she was 60. The doctor began to suffer from depression when she was in her training in anaesthetics and she writes, 'The evenings were the worst. I couldn't sleep; I woke up at 4 am. The hideous circuits of pain were particularly distressing at night. I resorted to sleeping tablets very early on in the illness. Without sleep I could not work; without work I had no hold on life, no direction, no future.' She goes on to describe her recovery and her effective treatment, but this took a considerable time to achieve. Some time after her recovery she was able to analyse the factors that had been important in bringing about a recovery and she lists them under seven factors all starting with the letter 'T'. The fifth 'T' is temazepam, and she writes, 'Temazepam – sleep was a relief from the pain in mind and body. I took no days off for the duration of the illness. I do not recommend such stoicism. Coping with mental illness is easier if sleep disturbance is corrected but medication must not be self prescribed; sick leave must be taken when necessary.'

Dr. Khursandi's account of the use of temazepam in conjunction with antidepressants is a good example of the importance of providing effective sleep in conjunction with antidepressant treatment. It is also an elegant example of the need to balance sensibly evidence-based medicine with valuable insights that can only be gleaned by sensitively treating individual patients and listening carefully to what they regard as important in aiding recovery and improvement.

3. Naturally, the use of benzodiazepines in short-term mild and moderate anxiety should be approached with caution but there is a role for these drugs in anxiety disorders. Despite the restrictive recommendations of the guidelines, many clinicians have continued to use these drugs.

The authors have continued to do this in their own clinical practice but using only a very small number of drugs – usually diazepam and chlordiazepoxide. However, on some occasions, the drug that the patient has already been started on by the family doctor is continued. On those occasions it is essential to keep in mind the equivalent strength of the various drugs because frequently the exact dose of the preparation is more relevant to the patient's exact requirements than the nature of the compound used. As this perspective is so important, the equivalent doses of these drugs (*British National Formulary*, 1999) are set out in Table 2.

Table 2. *Approximate equivalent doses of common benzodiazepines.*

Benzodiazepine	Oral dose	Equivalent diazepam dose
Chlordiazepoxide	15 mg	5 mg
Loprazolam	0.5–1 mg	5 mg
Lorazepam	500 μg	5 mg
Lormetazepam	0.5–1 mg	5 mg
Nitrazepam	5 mg	5 mg
Oxazepam	15 mg	5 mg
Temazepam	10 mg	5 mg

The great advantage to clinical practice is the obvious efficacy of diazepam and chlordiazepoxide in the treatment of anxiety and its related symptoms. The dose can be titrated easily so that symptom control can be accomplished without any reduction in alertness while the dose at night can be doubled to provide a much improved sleep pattern.

A distinct advantage of chlordiazepoxide is the virtual absence of any significant side effects when a dose of 10 mg is used. This fact can be conveyed fairly confidently to patients. If a patient does develop side effects then the chances are that the individual is a negative placebo responder and will have side effects with any prescribed medication.

Another reason for its use has been the existence for a long time of good quality evidence that at a dosage of 10 mg t.d.s. it is very unlikely to impair driving skills. A detailed study on police drivers in Basle (Kielholz *et al.*, 1967) provided good evidence of this.

THE WAY FORWARD

The natural history of a new drug can be divided into three distinct phases. The first is its introduction with publicity, even hype, and exaggerated expectation. The second phase is very different. New problems are identified and uncertainty develops about its role and usefulness. The third phase is the eventual resolution of the uncertainty about the new product by a clearer definition of the indications for its use, cautions, contraindications and side effects. Some drugs are abandoned completely. The debate over the benzodiazepines has never properly been resolved, with clinicians being divided into advocates, opponents and, perhaps, the majority, who use benzodiazepines with a degree of reluctance. It is now moving into a stage when the third phase can be spelt out with greater clarity.

To all those clinicians who had continued to use benzodiazepines for anxiety disorders, it was a great relief to read a comprehensive and scholarly review of the role of the benzodiazepines in anxiety disorders in the *New*

England Journal of Medicine in 1993 (Shader and Greenblatt, 1993). Not only was this paper published in a very prestigious journal but, in addition, the broad conclusions and recommendations that Shader and Greenblatt outlined resonated with the approach that had already been adopted by many clinicians. The conclusions of this paper can be regarded as a sound description of the continuing role of benzodiazepines in the management of anxiety disorders and it is worthwhile summarizing key parts of this paper.

- A careful review of the prescribing pattern in the USA already drew up a reassuring picture. It showed that the great majority of patients taking an anxiolytic drug take the medication for relatively short periods and only 15% of patients take it continuously for more that 1 year. In addition, the patients who take these drugs usually have high levels of emotional distress and have legitimate psychiatric diagnoses. The use of anxiolytic drugs in the USA has gradually decreased over time and the rate is similar in Western Europe and Canada. It was concluded that on balance the American public uses anti-anxiety agents conservatively and appropriately.
- Shader and Greenblatt considered that patients with symptoms of generalized anxiety disorder, which are not due to some other cause, should initially be considered for non-pharmacological treatment along with short-term counselling, psychotherapy, stress management, exercise and meditation. However, in many settings the availability of non-pharmacological treatment is limited and in these settings, pharmacological treatment may be the only option.
- In panic disorder, benzodiazepines reduce the frequency and severity of panic attacks and also the associated anticipatory anxiety and avoidance behaviour.
- The decision to prescribe a benzodiazepine should be based on the level of distress and level of functional disability, the potential hazards of non-treatment in relation to the probable success of pharmacological treatment and the hazards of medication. Initially, the longer-acting diazepam was more popular and then in the 1980s a shift towards using shorter acting drugs occurred. Nevertheless, trials comparing different benzodiazepines have failed to demonstrate a consistent difference in efficacy among the various drugs of this class.
- The approach to initiating treatment is based largely on clinical experience. A low-dose approach should be encouraged based on the patient's age, sex, body size, medication history and intensity of the clinical picture. The dose is increased gradually until the desired result is obtained or side effects intervene. The duration of drug treatment is tailored to the nature of the underlying illness and patients with intermittent symptoms can have intermittent therapy. Those with persisting, unremitting symptoms

may require more continuous treatment. However, the appropriate duration of treatment for such patients has not been clearly established.

- Some patients with anxiety or panic disorder may require indefinite treatment with benzodiazepines to live productive and comfortable lives. However, most patients should not receive continuous benzodiazepine therapy. Periodic reassessment of the need for medication makes clinical and medico-legal sense. After treatment for 4 months or less, the drug should be gradually discontinued. In some patients, the drug can be discontinued with no recurrence of symptoms. In other patients, symptoms recur during or after the period of withdrawal in which case therapy can be reinstituted. The strategy of periodic discontinuation should identify the subgroup of patients responsive to benzodiazepines whose anxiety is truly persistent and for whom long-term therapy may be beneficial. The size of this group is unknown and unfortunately there are no symptom criteria to identify these patients prospectively.

CONCLUSIONS

- The use of benzodiazepines in short-term, mild, generalized anxiety disorder should be approached with caution.
- In moderate and more severe states of generalized anxiety disorder, psychological approaches may be neither available nor appropriate. In these instances benzodiazepines are the safest drugs and invariably preferred by patients.
- A low-dose start should be coupled with dose titration to achieve effective symptom control.
- There is no evidence of the superiority of a particular benzodiazepine preparation.
- Length of treatment should be tailored to the pattern of illness. Intermittent symptoms may need intermittent therapy.
- Persisting and unremitting symptoms may require continuous treatment.
- A small number of patients may require indefinite treatment to live productive and comfortable lives. On these occasions periodic reassessment of the need of medication should be carried out.

REFERENCES

American Psychiatric Association (1994). *Diagnostic and Statistical Manual of Mental Disorder (4th edn)*. American Psychiatric Association, Washington, DC.

Berridge, V. (1999). *Opium and the People: Opiate Use and Drug Control Policy in Nineteenth Century England*. Free Association Books, London.

British National Formulary (1999). British Medical Association and Royal Pharmaceutical Society of Great Britain, London, p. 160.

Committee on Safety of Medicines (1988). Benzodiazepines, dependence and withdrawal symptoms. *Current Problems* **No. 21**, January 1988.

Khursandi, D.S. (1998). Personal View: Stars disappear. *BMJ* **317**, 480–481.

Kielholz, P., Goldberg, L., Obersteg, J., Poeldinger, W., Ramseyer, A., Schmidt, P. (1967). Strassenverker, Tranquilizer und Alcohol. *Dtsch Med Wochenschr* **92**, 1525–1531.

Lader, M. (1991). History of benzodiazepine dependence. *J Subst Abuse Treat* **8**, 53–59.

Oswald, I. (1986). Drugs for poor sleepers. *BMJ* **292**, 715.

Plant, M. (1999). Opium and the people: opiate use and drug control policy in nineteenth century England. *BMJ* **319**, 131.

Royal College of Psychiatrists (1988). Benzodiazepines and dependence: A College Statement. *Bull R Coll Psychiatr* **121**, 107–109.

Shader, R.I. and Greenblatt, D.J. (1993). Use of benzodiazepines in anxiety disorders. *N Engl J Med* **328**, 1398–1405.

Slater, E. and Roth, M. (1969). *Mayer-Gross, Slater and Roth Clinical Psychiatry (3rd edn)*. Baillière, Tindall & Cassell, London, pp. 415–416.

Williams, D.D.R. (1988). Use of benzodiazepines. *Bull R Coll Psychiatr* **8**, 453–454.

World Health Organization (1992). *The ICD-10 Classification of Mental and Behavioural Disorders* WHO, Geneva.

Benzodiazepines
Edited by Michael R. Trimble and Ian Hindmarch
Wrightson Biomedical Publishing Ltd
Chapter 5 © 2000 Crown copyright retained

5

Disturbed Sleep and Aviation Medicine

ANTHONY N. NICHOLSON

*Centre for Human Sciences, Defence Evaluation and Research Agency,
Farnborough, Hampshire, UK*

INTRODUCTION

Disturbed sleep is frequently encountered in the practice of aviation medicine – both with passengers and aircrew. Passengers have to cope with time zone changes after intercontinental flights; aircrew have to work at all times of the day and night, and those involved with long-haul flights also have to cope with time zone transitions. With both passengers and aircrew the question concerning the usefulness of hypnotics arises. In this chapter, the nature of sleep disturbance associated with air travel both for passengers and for aircrew will be described, and the management of aircrew coping with an irregular pattern of rest and of passengers who experience particular difficulty with intercontinental travel will be discussed.

NATURE OF SLEEP DISTURBANCE

Intercontinental travel

Sleep after an intercontinental flight is influenced by a variety of factors including the timing of the flight and the subsequent displacement of rest periods due to the direction of travel (Klein *et al.*, 1970, 1973; Nicholson *et al.*, 1986a). Westward flights across the North Atlantic involve a delay of 5–6 hours to the first rest period when individuals tend to fall asleep quickly and sleep more deeply. Clearly there is some degree of sleep deprivation, but falling asleep quickly is also related to the time of going to bed, which is well into the night of the natural rhythm for sleep and wakefulness. However,

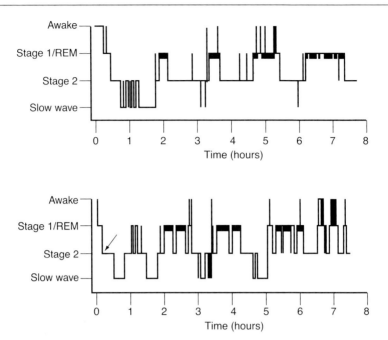

Figure 1. Control sleep recording (upper) and a hypnogram of the first night after a westward flight with a 5-hour time zone displacement (lower). The subject feel asleep quickly (arrow), but there was disturbed sleep during the latter half of the night.

sleep tends to be less restful during the latter part of the night as individuals try to continue sleeping until the local time of rising, which is around midday in the home time zone (Figure 1).

Delayed rest periods are also likely to modify the structure of sleep. The need for slow wave sleep will be stronger than usual during the early part of the night, and may reduce the amount of rapid eye movement (REM) activity that would be expected with individuals sleeping later in their rhythm of sleep and wakefulness. However, an increase in REM is likely to occur on the second night, when the need for slow wave sleep has subsided. By the third night after a westward flight the normal sleep pattern is usually well established. This indicates, together with the restoration to the usual time of day of the rising phase of the circadian rhythm of alertness, that the individual, at least as far as his or her sleep–wakefulness continuum is concerned, has adapted to the new time zone.

In the case of eastward journeys across the North Atlantic, sleep during the first night may be even better than before the flight as passengers may not have slept on the aircraft or even during the first day in the new time zone. However, in the new time zone, with an advance of the sleep period, sleep

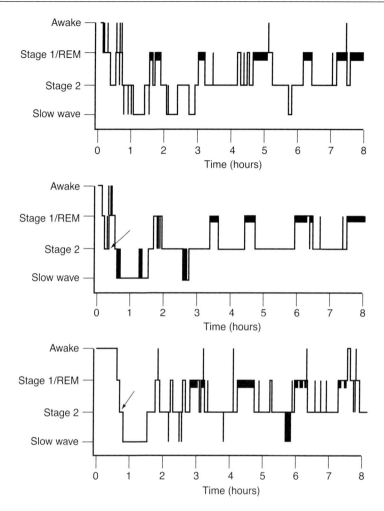

Figure 2. Control sleep recording (upper) and a hypnogram of the first (middle) and fifth (lower) nights after an eastward flight with a 5-hour time zone displacement. The subject did not sleep during the overnight flight and so sleep onset during the first night in the new time zone (19-hour delay) was quick (arrow) and well sustained. During the fifth night, sleep onset was slow (arrow), and there were many awakenings.

onset is delayed once the immediate effect of sleep loss is overcome (Figure 2). An advance in the period of sleep is also likely to reduce REM activity. For several nights after eastward journeys slow wave sleep, total sleep time and sleep efficiency are reduced and there are more awakenings. Eventually, on the fourth, fifth or sixth night, there is an increase in REM to compensate for the REM deficit that has accumulated, and thereafter sleep returns to normal. These changes, together with the slow realignment of the normal pattern of daytime alertness, show that the sleep–wakefulness continuum may not relate to local time for several days after an eastward flight.

The greater difficulty in adapting to an eastward than to a westward transition is a reflection of the speed of resynchronization of the underlying circadian rhythm. A partial explanation of this is that our innate circadian rhythmicity is longer than the day–night cycle, and that without the influence of the environment there is a natural tendency to lengthen the day. This is the tendency after a westward flight with its delay to sleep, but after an eastward flight we have to shorten our day and there may be an inherent resistance. Thus, after a long eastward transition some individuals may actually prefer to lengthen their day in the process of adaptation. As far as aircrew are concerned, long eastward transitions are among the most disruptive. As well as sleep disturbance, which can last for at least 6 days, levels of alertness during the day may be impaired for a similar period. The reasons for the extent of this disturbance are not fully understood, but they may be related to the large reduction in amplitude of the circadian rhythm that usually coincides with rapid changes in phase.

The main problem with transmeridian flights is coping with, rather than adapting to, a time zone change (Nicholson *et al.*, 1986b; Wegmann *et al.*, 1986). After a westward flight passengers usually sleep well, even though there may be somewhat less restful sleep in the latter half of the night. The timing of the eastward return flight is important, particularly if it is overnight. In a visit of a day or two, some shift of the circadian rhythm to the new local time will have taken place, though the period of maximum alertness may still occur earlier than if the rhythm was fully synchronized. During the day of this return flight eastward, individuals may be less alert than usual during the late afternoon and early evening. In this event, a departure around 18.00 could follow a nap in the afternoon – particularly useful for aircrew operating overnight. The advance of the phase of the alertness rhythm relative to the home time zone would ensure increasing alertness during the latter part of the flight terminating during the early morning. It can be seen that correct timing of flights may have many advantages for aircrew.

Irregularity of working hours

The sleep patterns of aircrew are seriously disturbed by repeated crossing of time zones, as in worldwide operations (Nicholson, 1970), or repeated night flights, as during intercontinental north–south operations. In these circumstances sleep patterns are irregular, and sleep disturbance may persist for several days after schedules that include repeated transmeridian flights. The sleep of aircrew operating an eastward round-the-world schedule is illustrated in Figure 3. Irregularity of sleep both with respect to duration and

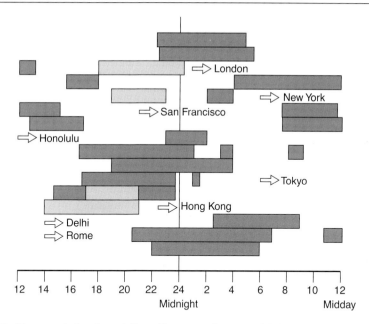

Figure 3. Sleep periods of an airline pilot operating a worldwide east–west schedule (Nicholson, 1970). The figure is read from the bottom line up, and each line is from midday of one day to midday the next; each rectangle is a period of sleep and hatched rectangles indicate subjectively poor sleep. Arrows indicate commencement of duty.

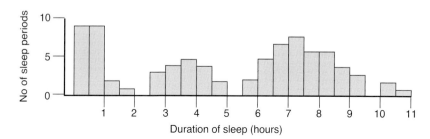

Figure 4. Frequency of sleep periods of various durations over a month for a pilot operating worldwide routes. Sleep periods of around 1 hour are naps, whereas periods of around 3–4 hours are often anticipatory sleeps.

time of day is evident. Indeed, the dominant feature of the sleep of aircrew who operate worldwide routes is irregularity, in terms of both duration of sleep and the time of day when it occurs (Figure 4).

Adaptation of the sleep of aircrew operating worldwide east–west routes has received much attention. When the rest period is 24 hours, a long sleep immediately after a flight could mean that the crew may not be in the most rested state possible during the next duty period commencing 12 hours after the end of the sleep period. To avoid undue sleepiness during duty after a 24-hour rest, crews often split their sleep into two parts. The need for sleep immediately before duty (an anticipatory sleep) is created by restricting sleep immediately after the preceding flight. This often leads to sleep periods of 3–4 hours during long-haul schedules. During flights that extend wakefulness beyond 16 hours and flights that start during the early evening, naps of 30 minutes to 1 hour are not uncommon, and they are clearly useful during westward flights when the day is lengthened (Figure 4).

Short periods of sleep are taken to maintain effectiveness during schedules that include irregularity of rest. However, although naps of about an hour decrease the tendency to sleep, it would appear they have a less beneficial effect on performance when an individual is already impaired – as during a long overnight duty period. On the other hand, periods of sleep of about 4 hours taken before overnight work can be very useful. Levels of performance fall precipitously when the end of a long period of work coincides with the fall in performance associated with the circadian rhythm of the individual, but with a 4-hour period of sleep during the evening (anticipatory sleep) there can be a sustained improvement in performance over the night (Nicholson *et al.*, 1985). Performance overnight may be more easily sustained by a preceding sleep of several hours than by attempting to overcome the effects of sleep loss by a nap. Sleep preceding long duty periods is a useful strategy.

Careful attention to sleep is undoubtedly important when rest periods are irregularly placed – as with long-haul aircrew. Impaired performance follows sleep disturbance, even though the impairment is not always easy to demonstrate. Sleep disturbance modifies circadian functions, impairs response to stress and upsets the normal sense of well-being. Essentially, the measurement of behaviour is insufficiently sophisticated to detect change in many important functions, and this has tended to further the myth that disturbed sleep has limited import. This is not so. Performance is maintained by greater effort or by concentrating attention on limited aspects of the problem for a limited period of time, while interpersonal skills, judgement and decision-making may be impaired.

MANAGEMENT OF SLEEP DISTURBANCE

Passengers

The most useful approach for passengers embarking upon an intercontinental flight is to travel at the right time of day. There is a simple piece of advice for the intercontinental traveller: *Travel west, travel later; travel east, travel earlier.* In both cases – if the schedule is arranged correctly – the passenger would arrive in time for bed. For the transatlantic trip, an aircraft at 17.00 to New York arriving at 20.00 local time would be ideal. On the other hand, when travelling from New York to London a morning flight would be ideal. With 'loss' of several hours of time arrival would be late in the evening. Of course, there are not always services available to meet itineraries, but increasing availability and choice does make planning more possible.

Avoiding travel overnight, if at all possible, is a useful initial approach, but, then, there is the need to establish bodily rhythms to the final destination. Difficulty in adjusting sleep is likely to be met by all passengers from time to time, and adjustment itself needs time. Many years ago, the International Civil Aviation Organization devised a formula to determine the amount of rest needed after intercontinental travel. It was based on several factors: the duration of the journey (for travel itself can be fatiguing); the number of time zones; and the time of departure or arrival. In the case of travel from Montreal to Mexico, no particular period of rest was prescribed, whereas with travel from Montreal to Lima about 1½ days of rest was recommended, particularly with a departure at 15.00. Transatlantic travel depended on the direction and also on the time of departure. Leaving Montreal at 21.00 would require a day of rest in London, but leaving London at 15.00 would not require any rest on arrival in Montreal. With travel beyond the North Atlantic the picture was different. Leaving Montreal at 23.00 for Karachi would require 2½ days to recover, and leaving Montreal for Sydney at 10.00 would also require a similar period of recovery time.

Aircrew

The approach to the complaint of sleep difficulty in aircrew is much more complex, and it has to be based on the individual's history and medical details, and on specialized investigations. Difficulties related to rest being taken at unusual times and to the circumstances that surround rest not being conducive to sleep (transient insomnia) are likely to be the presenting complaint of aircrew. However, it must be borne in mind that a history of sleep disturbance over several weeks (short-term insomnia) is more likely to be related to a life crisis or a medical illness rather than to work. The irregularity of rest superimposed upon sleep of poor quality can be very troublesome and so a careful assessment of sleep should always be made in aircrew, particularly in middle-aged staff, who complain of persistent difficulty in coping with their work.

Difficulties experienced by aircrew in coping with their schedules may involve other factors, but an important aspect to successful management is undoubtedly proper arrangements for duty. Disturbed sleep may arise from long-haul operations, which involve complete irregularity of work and rest, and from short-haul schedules, which encroach on the beginning and the end of the sleep period over many months. Sleep disturbance could prejudice the safety of air operations, and so workload must allow crews to achieve acceptable sleep. The scheduling of duty, particularly as aircrew have to remain continuously on task, must avoid marked falls in performance due to the adverse juxtaposition of prolonged duty (time on task) with the nadir of circadian rhythm performance (time of day). Such considerations are intended to be embodied in flight time limitations, though these do not necessarily lead to schedules acceptable to all aircrew.

In the initial consultation, the practitioner must explore the possibility of a background of recent sleep disturbance which may reflect personal difficulties, either at home or at work, or a history over many months or years which would raise the question of chronic insomnia or a sleep disorder. The decision of whether polysomnography is a necessary part of the assessment will depend on the information gained, and, perhaps, any subsequent response to sleep counselling, but it is usually an essential investigation in aircrew with persistent or recurrent sleep difficulty. Narcolepsy and the delayed phase syndrome must be borne in mind in younger aircrew, and in middle-aged aircrew the normal deterioration of sleep may be exaggerated by apnoeas and leg movements. Such events in themselves may have limited or no clinical significance, but they could imply obstructive sleep apnoea or be a manifestation of the restless legs syndrome.

If the practitioner is satisfied that there is no significant medical or behavioural background to the complaint and that the individual is free of a sleep disorder, the initial approach is to counsel the individual to look after their sleep both at home and at work. Attention to sleep habits is essential for all patients with a sleep problem. Indeed, poor sleep hygiene is always either the cause or a contributory factor, and so is important to the management of sleep difficulties. In the initial investigation, a diary details of the pattern of sleep and wakefulness will prove most valuable. It is important that the data covers the patterns of work and rest both at home and when on duty, and should cover several weeks. Careful appraisal of this information will give important leads to the main cause of sleep difficulties.

HYPNOTICS

Real difficulty in sleep in passengers and aircrew free of a background problem in insomnia or sleep disorder, and after attention to sleep habits, raises the question of the occasional use of hypnotics. In both passengers and aircrew, the difficulty is a transient one with unequivocal evidence of disturbed sleep, and so the judicious use of a hypnotic is warranted. The prescribed hypnotic must be appropriate to the problem and this means that the normal architecture of sleep must not be disturbed both during the time of treatment and on withdrawal, and that the drug itself is free of unwanted effects during subsequent daytime vigilance.

In the practice of aviation medicine, the most significant property of a hypnotic (for both passengers and aircrew) is its duration of action, and this depends on absorption, distribution and elimination. The rate of absorption determines onset of action because hypnotics penetrate the blood–brain barrier with ease. Rapid absorption is associated with quick onset of action whereas with slow absorption the desired effect may be attenuated or even absent. A peak plasma level around an hour after ingestion is essential. After absorption a hypnotic is distributed to the blood and to highly vascular tissues. The initial fall in the plasma concentration may be quite marked, and this relates primarily to this distribution phase. The latter part of the fall relates to elimination by metabolism and by excretion. In general, because hypnotics cross the blood–brain barrier with ease, a drug has an effect as long as its plasma concentration remains above a certain level. The duration of action will be short if this level is within the phase that predominantly represents distribution, but if the level is within an elimination phase that is slower than the distribution phase, it may be much longer. Rapid elimination of parent compounds and of metabolites is, therefore, essential to ensure freedom from daytime effects.

Experience extending nearly 30 years in the UK in both military and civil aviation has led to temazepam 10–20 mg being the drug of choice for aircrew, but it is important to use a rapidly absorbed formulation. It is equally useful for passengers. Temazepam has a short duration of action due to its predominant distribution phase, and its rate of elimination is such that a single dose is free of residual effects. Its short duration of action provides an adequate margin of safety for use by aircrew during demanding schedules. It is unfortunate that the misuse of temazepam has necessitated strict control of this hypnotic, and so it is not so easily prescribed as previously. Although the administrative inconvenience of prescribing temazepam should not have an overriding influence on its use in aviation, it may well be that it will be replaced by a hypnotic of similar pharmacokinetic properties; zolpidem is a clear candidate.

Any hypnotics with which the practitioner and the passenger or crew are unfamiliar should tried 'on the ground' before being prescribed for use during schedules. It should then be given at the lowest dose and as infrequently as possible. In the use of hypnotics *en route*, the practitioner should help to identify when it is likely to be most beneficial. For aircrew there should be an interval of 24 hours between ingestion and commencement of duty, though under supervision the interval may be reduced to 12 hours. Perhaps it is unnecessary to emphasize that if hypnotics are to be used in the management of sleep disturbance in aircrew the use of alcohol should be limited and preferably avoided.

A short-acting hypnotic such as temazepam (10–20 mg) should always be used by aircrew, but with passengers the overriding issue is adaptation to a new time zone rather than to ensure adequate sleep within a limited period of rest. In this context a slightly longer-acting hypnotic may be more useful. Brotizolam (0.25 mg) is an excellent hypnotic to ensure sleep after a time zone transition and is without residual impairment of performance. An alternative, zolpidem (10 mg), is also free of residual effects. Some hypnotics such as zopiclone have residual effects on performance if used in the recommended dose range (3.75–7.5 mg).

SUMMARY

In the management of sleep disturbance inevitable with worldwide air travel, it is essential, in the first place, to understand how the disturbance arises and the nature of the changes in sleep. In both passengers and aircrew, these are the primary considerations from which appropriate management can be planned. Hypnotics are a useful adjunct. They are particularly helpful for passengers adapting to eastward transitions and for aircrew having to cope with irregular periods of work. With passengers the main consideration is usually the need to sustain sleep in the new time zone. The usefulness of a hypnotic for aircrew is largely dependent on whether it possesses the pharmacokinetic profile to ensure a rapid onset of sleep and freedom from residual effects at the end of a rest period of limited duration.

REFERENCES

Klein, K.E., Bruner, H., Holtmann, H., Rehme, H., Stolze, H., Steinhoff, W.D. and Wegmann, H.M. (1970). Circadian rhythm of pilots' efficiency and effects of multiple time zone travel. *Aerospace Med* **41**, 125–132.

Klein, K.E., Wegmann, H.M. and Hunt, J.B. (1973). Desynchronisation of body temperature and performance circadian rhythms as a result of outgoing and homecoming transmeridian flights. *Aerospace Med* **43**, 119–132.

Nicholson, A.N. (1970). Sleep patterns of an airline pilot operating world-wide east–west routes. *Aerospace Med* **41**, 626–632.

Nicholson, A.N., Pascoe, P.A., Roehrs, T., Roth, T., Spencer, M.B., Stone, B.M. and Zorick, F. (1985). Sustained performance with short evening and morning sleeps. *Aviat Space Environ Med* **56**, 105–114.

Nicholson, A.N., Pascoe, P.A., Spencer, M.B., Stone, B.M., Roehrs, T. and Roth, T. (1986a). Sleep after transmeridian flights. *Lancet* **ii**, 1205–1208.

Nicholson, A.N., Pascoe, P.A., Spencer, M.B., Stone, B.M. and Green, R.L. (1986b). Nocturnal sleep and daytime alertness of aircrew after transmeridian flights. *Aviat Space Environ Med* **57**, B42–B52.

Wegmann, H.M., Gundel, A., Naumann, M., Samel, A., Schwartz, E. and Vejvoda, M. (1986). Sleep, sleepiness and circadian rhythmicity in aircrews operating transatlantic routes. *Aviat Space Environ Med* **57**, B53–B64.

Benzodiazepines
Edited by Michael R. Trimble and Ian Hindmarch
© 2000 Wrightson Biomedical Publishing Ltd

6

Benzodiazepines in Epilepsy: An Overview

MICHAEL R. TRIMBLE

Raymond Way Neuropsychiatry Unit, Institute of Neurology, London, UK

INTRODUCTION

The benzodiazepines are amongst the most powerful antiepileptic that are available. Ever since their introduction in the 1970s they have found a place in the management of patients with epilepsy, particularly in status epilepticus, but also in the management of refractory cases. Their use has been reviewed in a number of texts, most recently by Ko and colleagues (1997). There are two main groups in clinical practice: the 1,4-benzodiazepines and the 1,5-benzodiazepines. The numbering refers to the nitrogen substitution in either the fourth or fifth position of the diazepam ring. They almost certainly work in epilepsy by activation of gamma-aminobutyric acid (GABA)-A receptors, leading in the cell to the acceleration inward of chloride molecules, resulting in cell membrane hyperpolarization.

BENZODIAZEPINES FOR THE MANAGEMENT OF EPILEPSY

A number of compounds, reviewed by Walker and Sander (see Chapter 7), are used to control status epilepticus, including diazepam, clonazepam and midazolam. With regard to oral treatment, the most popularly used drugs are clonazepam, clorazepate, nitrazepam and clobazam.

Clonazepam has been shown to have a wide efficacy in both partial and generalized seizures (Browne, 1978) and is used mainly as adjunctive therapy for patients with resistant primary and secondary generalized seizures. It is in addition used in difficult to control absence seizures, myoclonic seizures and post-anoxic cerebellar myoclonus. It has been successfully prescribed for the management of juvenile myoclonic epilepsy and some of the progressive hereditary myoclonic syndromes.

Clorazepate, the prodrug of desmethyldiazepam, is likewise used as add-on therapy for a variety of resistant seizures, although both the data and the use of this product are rather less than for clonazepam.

Nitrazepam tends to be used in paediatric epilepsy, but again covering a variety of seizure types such as infantile spasms, myoclonic seizures and the Lennox–Gastaut syndrome.

The above compounds are all 1,4-benzodiazepines. While there are reports of some others from this group, such as lorazepam and chlordiazepoxide, also being used in the oral therapy of resistant epilepsy, they have never found any particular niche.

The 1,4-benzodiazepines are acknowledged to have two main problems when it comes to the management of chronic epilepsy: the first is sedation, and the second is the development of tolerance. Tolerance is discussed in a later chapter (see Chapter 9), but it is well known that patients often respond well initially to an oral benzodiazepine, only to find that the major effect wears off after a few weeks. The mechanism of tolerance is unknown, and whether or not it is similar to the mechanism of the tolerance that can be generated to the anxiolytic effects of these drugs is not clear. However, it is known that some of the 1,4-benzodiazepines can lead to drug dependence, and that withdrawal symptoms (including seizures) can occur following cessation of these drugs, which must, in most cases, be undertaken slowly.

THE 1,5-BENZODIAZEPINES

The 1,5-benzodiazepines appear to have a benefit over the 1,4-benzodiazepines of being less sedative and having a wider therapeutic index. The only 1,5-benzodiazepine available for oral treatment is clobazam. It was introduced to the UK in 1979, and since that time has found wide use in a number of different seizure types – a subject that has been extensively reviewed (Robertson, 1995).

Following an oral dose, peak plasma levels of clobazam occur within 3 hours of administration; the half-life of clobazam itself is a mean of 18 hours (range of 10–30 hours). Clobazam has a number of metabolites, but the main one, N-desmethylclobazam, has a half-life in the range of 60 hours, which is considerably longer than that of the parent compound. In long-term administration, the plasma levels of N-desmethylclobazam become greater than those of clobazam, and thus the anticonvulsant properties of clobazam are at least in part attributable to this metabolite.

CLINICAL STUDIES OF CLOBAZAM

Clinical studies of clobazam have been reviewed by Robertson (1995). There are seven double-blind and one single-blind study in the literature, each demonstrating the efficacy of the compound in comparison with placebo. The drug was used as add-on therapy and the patients were typical for these kind of studies, namely those with intractable seizures that have not responded to first- or second-line treatment. The exception to this was the study by Feely and colleagues (1982) in which the drug was used intermittently to treat catamenial seizures (see Chapter 10).

The largest database was the European multicentre investigation of Koeppen and colleagues (1987) who compared clobazam and placebo in 129 treatment-resistant patients, 89% of whom had complex partial seizures. The trial duration was 7 months, with two 3-month treatment periods and a 1-month switch over. The dose of clobazam ranged from 10 to 40 mg a day. A significant reduction in seizures was noted in the active treatment group: 19% of patients receiving clobazam became seizure-free during the treatment period. No patient became seizure-free on placebo.

In addition to these trials, there are 35 open studies of clobazam looking at the effects of the drug in a similar population group. These cover a total of 2259 patients, ages ranging from 4 months to 84 years, with all types of seizures. Within these studies, three were of clobazam given as monotherapy in children.

Robertson (1995) reported that the overall effect of the reduction of seizure frequency with clobazam was 65%, although it was difficult to be certain because of the differing seizure classifications that various authors had used to monitor change. She reported that 28 of the studies reported on complete cessation of seizures, with a total of 18% becoming attack-free.

Another large study was by the Canadian Clobazam Co-operative group (1991). They had 877 patients, but the study was retrospective. Over half of the patients were children, and a number of these were learning disabled. In this study, the duration of the clobazam therapy was from days to 4 years, but more than 40% of patients were treated for more than 1 year. It was interesting to note that 4 years after starting the drug, nearly half of the patients were continuing to take clobazam, and that 40% of patients reported significant clinical improvement in their seizures. At the time of the study, over 8% of patients were seizure-free.

FREEDOM OF SEIZURES WITH CLOBAZAM

One of the most important goals of managing epilepsy is to render a patient seizure-free. It is known that with well-adjusted monotherapy some 60–70%

of patients will achieve this goal, but it is the 30–40% who continue to have seizures in spite of the use of standardized antiepileptic drugs with good serum level monitoring where recurrent seizures persist who require adjunctive therapy. It is to this group that the challenge for new antiepileptic drugs has emerged.

However, from the clinical trials of new antiepileptic drugs it is often difficult to ascertain the percentage of patients with adjunctive therapy who become seizure-free. Some compounds, such as vigabatrin, appear to give a seizure freedom rate of between 7% and 10%, this drug probably being the most powerful of all of the newly introduced treatments. Clobazam stands up well in this regard (for references see Robertson, 1995). Although the studies quoted contain some of the earlier clinical trials, it does seem to be the case that patients can remain seizure-free on clobazam following long-term follow-up, and that only a subgroup of patients develop tolerance. In the study by Reynolds and colleagues (Heller *et al.* 1988), 41 patients with resistant epilepsy were given clobazam as adjunctive therapy. 40% were seizure-free. The data from the Canadian Clobazam Co-operation group (1991) showed that if patients continued taking clobazam, 21% were seizure-free. During the first month, 60% of patients had dramatic improvements in their seizure frequency, but this fell to 30% at 6 months, and 20% at 1 year. However, importantly, after a year of treatment, 10% of patients remained seizure-free. Similar figures for seizure freedom were given following long-term treatment (over 12 months) by Guberman and colleagues (1990) (10%) and Wolf (1985) (17%).

SIDE EFFECTS

One of the major advantages of the 1,5-benzodiazepine clobazam is that it appears to have much less in the way of sedative properties than the 1,4-benzodiazepines. This has been demonstrated in a number of human psychopharmacological investigations where in addition to anxiolytic properties, the drug has been shown if anything to possess mild psychoactive properties. This includes, in particular, an effect on the Critical Flicker Fusion threshold in an opposite direction to the standard benzodiazepines.

Thus, in epilepsy, clobazam is well tolerated, and minimal side effects are usually reported. The main ones relate to adverse mood changes and tiredness, which are common to all of the benzodiazepines. The mood changes include irritability, dysphoria and sometimes aggressive episodes; rarer reported treatment emergent effects include hyperkinesis, anorexia, an increase in seizure frequency, and psychosis. The latter can occur as the phenomenon of forced normalization, in which a psychosis can emerge in patients with chronic seizures who suddenly have their seizure suppressed by the administration of an effective anticonvulsant (Trimble and Schmitz, 1998). In these patients, the electroencephalogram loses its previous interictal epileptic discharges, effectively becoming 'more normal'. The psychoses are seen following administration of a number of antiepileptic compounds that effectively prevent seizures occurring, and should to a large extent be seen as a seizure-related phenomenon.

Not surprisingly, side effects from clobazam are seen more frequently when the drug is used in polytherapy compared with monotherapy, particularly when levels of N-desmethylclobazam reach over about 5 µg/ml.

These data are complemented by many reports of a general improvement of behaviour in patients treated with clobazam (for full review see Robertson, 1995). In a comparative study, clobazam (10 mg three times a day) was compared with clonazepam (0.5 mg three times a day) in a crossover study of healthy volunteers where the benzodiazepines were compared with placebo. The active drug and the placebo were given for 2 weeks. Psychological performance was monitored using computer-given psychological tests, and the results showed only minimal impairment of cognitive function with clobazam in comparison with clonazepam, which affected a broad spectrum of cognitive abilities (Cull and Trimble, 1985).

Willden and colleagues (1990) also compared clobazam with clonazepam, also using healthy volunteers, although the drug was given for only brief periods. In this study, 10 mg and 20 mg of clobazam produced fewer psychomotor side effects than 0.5 mg and 1 mg of clonazepam.

WITHDRAWAL PHENOMENON

As with most antiepileptic drugs, and as with other benzodiazepines, the problem of withdrawal seizures with clobazam is important clinically. The fact that N-desmethylclobazam has such a long half-life is probably one reason why there is little chance of any psychological withdrawal symptoms emerging after use with clobazam, as indeed the literature suggests. However, because withdrawal seizures are encountered in a number of the clinical trials, it is considered wise to withdraw clobazam slowly, if necessary taking several months.

RECOMMENDED USE OF CLOBAZAM IN EPILEPSY

There is no intravenous preparation available; clobazam use is therefore as adjunctive oral therapy. It has been used in a monotherapy setting, and most practitioners have experience of patients who have become seizure-free on clobazam and can then slowly be withdrawn from their existing therapy.

The advantages of clobazam have been outlined by Guberman (1995) as follows:

- it is a broad spectrum anticonvulsant
- it can be given once or twice a day because of its long half-life
- it is effective in refractive patients
- it has a high therapeutic index with a rapid onset of action
- it has an anxiolytic effect
- there are few drug interactions
- there are no enzyme-inducing effects
- there are no serious adverse consequences of the drug
- there is no evidence of abuse.

The drug is usually considered as adjunctive therapy in epilepsy; essentially the indication for clobazam is therefore for use in patients who have failed to respond to standard antiepileptic drug treatment, using effective serum level monitoring.

This brings us into the realm of polytherapy. The literature and clinical practice have for many years encouraged treatment with monotherapy. However, since the introduction of a host of new antiepileptic drugs we are now back in an era of unbridled polypharmacy. Sometimes this is politely referred to as rational polypharmacy, but it certainly is the case that many patients with difficult to control seizures are now receiving several of the newer compounds, all of which powerfully affect central nervous system activity. In a patient with intractable epilepsy, the options for further management include reviewing the diagnosis. It is well acknowledged that many patients with intractable seizures may not have epilepsy at all (perhaps up to 20% in chronic epilepsy clinics), and re-review of the patient's history and seizure pattern may suggest an alternative diagnosis, in particular pseudoseizures.

Further, it is clear that the option to have surgical treatment, in particular a temporal lobectomy, is still widely underused. This is a highly effective method of managing patients with epilepsy (rendering some 70% seizure-free), although this can only be done after extensive and expensive investigation.

Following consideration of those options, one of the newer antiepileptic drugs is then given as adjunctive therapy. (How many of these new agents should be used before an option for surgery is investigated is quite unclear. However, trials with all of the new drugs could take several years, by which time the chances of successful surgery may have declined.)

There are no hard and fast rules about which drugs to use. There are reasons to prefer one compound over another: this may depend on the seizure type (for example vigabatrin for infantile spasms); a desire to minimize pharmacokinetic interactions (for example with gabapentin); or a desire to seek a pharmacodynamic interaction which may be clinically beneficial (for example between lamotrigine and sodium valproate). There are, however, also economic consequences of prescribing these new agents (see Chapter 12), and then there are purely pragmatic reasons – some physicians preferring one drug to another because of greater experience.

With regard to the benzodiazepines, it seems clear that they have stood the test of time to have a place in oral therapy for epilepsy as well as in status epilepticus. However, with regard to oral therapy, few compounds have been widely used, clobazam and clonazepam being preferred choices. There are clear differences between these drugs: evidence suggests that clobazam has less side effects and a better therapeutic profile.

If clobazam is to be used as adjunctive therapy, it is logical to give it before some of the other newer compounds, not only on economic grounds, but also because of its safety profile. Although the problem with tolerance is clear, it seems to be the case that tolerance can be seen with many of these compounds. More important is the fact that a long-term response is seen in some 40–60% of patients who are given clobazam, and that about 10% will remain seizure-free after a year or more of treatment.

The usual dose is to start with 10 mg of clobazam, although recently 5 mg tablets have been introduced, and particularly in children this is a preferable initial step. It is possible to give the drug as a single night-time dose, enhancing compliance and minimizing any possible sedative effects that the drug might induce.

In addition to its use as add-on therapy, clobazam has been particularly useful in the management of patients with intermittent bouts of seizures, including clusters and catamenial seizures. With regard to clusters, these can sometimes herald the onset of a post-ictal behaviour disturbance, including post-ictal psychosis. One useful effect of clobazam is therefore to give it to patients to take (or to their relatives to administer) following the first seizure of what might become a cluster, with 10 mg being given every 6 hours for 48 hours. This is useful not only in preventing the cluster from evolving, but also in preventing the later onset of the psychosis. Similarly, clobazam has been used for the prophylaxis of recurrent febrile convulsions, particularly when there is a reluctance to give rectal diazepam. There are reports of clobazam being used beneficially in patients with repeated bouts of non-convulsive status epilepticus (Gubermann, 1995), with doses of 50 mg or 60 mg being given when the status epilepticus begins; some patients seemingly responding to clobazam when other treatments including intravenous diazepam have not been of value.

Clobazam is particularly useful in the paediatric setting, having been introduced, some 20 years ago, for the treatment of the Lennox–Gastaut syndrome by Henri Gastaut himself.

CONCLUSIONS

The benzodiazepines have a useful role to play in the management of patients with intractable seizures, in addition to their value as first-line management for status epilepticus. As oral therapy, several of them have been used over the years, but at the present time the most commonly prescribed are clonazepam and clobazam. There are differences in the profiles of these drugs, particularly from the point of view of adverse effects, and this chapter has reviewed mainly the role of clobazam as adjunctive therapy for patients with difficult to control epilepsy in a variety of clinical settings. It appears to have a good clinical effect, tolerance and tiredness being the two main side effects, but is generally well tolerated by patients. Its pharmacokinetics, pharmacodynamics and safety profile have been accumulated after many years of experience with the drug.

REFERENCES

Browne, T.R. (1978). Clonazepam. *N Engl J Med* **299**, 812–816.

Canadian Clobazam Co-operative Group (1991). Clobazam in the treatment of refractory epilepsy: the Canadian experience. A retrospective study. *Epilepsia* **32**, 407–416.

Cull, C. and Trimble, M.R. (1985). Anticonvulsant benzodiazepines and performance. In: Hindmarch, I., Stonier, P.D. and Trimble, M.R. (Eds), *Clobazam: Human Psychopharmacology and Clinical Applications.* Royal Society of Medicine, London, pp. 121–128.

Feely, M., Calvert, T.R. and Gibson, J. (1982). Clobazam in catamenial epilepsy: a model for evaluating anticonvulsants. *Lancet* **ii**, 71–73.

Guberman, A.H. (1995). Adjunctive therapy with benzodiazepines. *Hum Psychopharmacol* **10**, S75–77.

Gubermann, A. Couture, M., Blaschuk, K. and Sherwin, A. (1990). Add-on trial of clobazam in intractable adult epilepsy with plasma level correlations. *Can J Neuro Sci* **17**, 311–316.

Heller, A.J., Ring, H.A. and Reynolds, E.H. (1988). Factors relating to dramatic response to clobazam therapy in refractory epilepsy. *Epilepsy Res* **2**, 276–280.

Ko, D.Y., Rho, J.M., De Giorgio, C.M. and Sato, S. (1997). Benzodiazepines. In: Engel, J. and Pedley, T.A. (Eds), *Epilepsy: A Comprehensive Textbook.* Raven Press, Philadelphia, pp. 1475–1489.

Koeppen, D., Baruzzi, A., Capozza, M. *et al.* (1987). Clobazam in therapy resistant patients with partial epilepsy: a double blind placebo controlled cross over study. *Epilepsia* **28**, 495–506.

Robertson, M.M. (1995). The place of Clobazam in the treatment of epilepsy: an update. *Hum Psychopharmacol* **10**, S43–63.

Trimble, M.R. and Schmitz, B. (1998). *Forced Normalisation and Alternative Psychoses of Epilepsy.* Wrightson Biomedical Press, Petersfield, Hants.

Willden, J.N., Pleuvery, B.J., Bawer, G.E., Onon, T. and Millington, L. (1990). Respiratory and sedative effects of clobazam and clonazepam in volunteers. *Br J Clin Pharmacol* **29**, 169–177.

Wolf, P. (1985). Clobazam in drug resistant patients with complex focal seizures. In: Hindmarch, I., Stonier, P.D. and Trimble, M.R. (Eds), *Clobazam: Human Psychopharmacology and Clinical Applications.* Royal Society of Medicine, London, pp. 167–171.

Benzodiazepines
Edited by Michael R. Trimble and Ian Hindmarch
© 2000 Wrightson Biomedical Publishing Ltd

7

Benzodiazepines in Status Epilepticus

M.C. WALKER and J.W. SANDER

University Department of Clinical Neurology, Institute of Neurology, London, UK

INTRODUCTION

Seizures are for the most part self-terminating. On occasions, however, seizures of any type can continue unabated and they are then considered as a separate entity, status epilepticus. In the nineteenth century, status epilepticus was clearly distinguished amongst the epilepsies. Calmeil (1824) used the term *état de mal* and later the term status epilepticus appeared in Bazire's translation of Trousseau's lectures on clinical medicine. From that time status epilepticus was, on the whole, a term used to describe solely convulsive status epilepticus. It was not until the Marseilles conference in 1962 that status epilepticus was recognized to include all seizure types and that its definition was based solely on the persistence of the seizure rather than its form (Gastaut *et al.*, 1967). Status epilepticus was defined as 'a condition characterised by epileptic seizures that are sufficiently prolonged or repeated at sufficiently brief intervals so as to produce an unvarying and enduring epileptic condition' (Gastaut, 1973). This definition is vague and to some extent inaccurate because status epilepticus is best viewed as a varying condition, as will be discussed. There has also been debate concerning the time period that fulfils the criterion of 'sufficiently prolonged'. Thirty minutes of seizure activity is generally taken as the definition of status epilepticus; treatment, however, should probably begin after 5 minutes of continuous convulsive seizure activity because after this period it is unlikely that the seizure will self-terminate (Lowenstein *et al.*, 1999).

The term status epilepticus included three entities: generalized status epilepticus; partial status epilepticus; and unilateral status epilepticus (Gastaut *et al.*, 1967). This classification is, however, both incomplete and too broad to be clinically useful, and further more detailed electroclinical classifications have been proposed. Shorvon (1994) classified status epilepticus according to the age at which it occurred, but once again this classification fails in that it does not describe the underlying aetiology, which in many cases is the major determinant of prognosis.

Status epilepticus is a relatively common condition. In a prospective study in Richmond, Virginia (DeLorenzo et al., 1996), the overall incidence was estimated as 41–61 per 100 000 person-years with a mortality of 9–17 per 100 000 person-years. Overall, 13.3% had recurrent attacks, 58% had no previous history of epilepsy and the mortality was 22%. Elderly people had the highest incidence of attacks with the greatest mortality (38%) and the least history of prior epilepsy (30%). Although the prognosis of status epilepticus was related to aetiology, the prognosis of certain conditions such as stroke appeared to be very much worse if they were associated with status epilepticus than if they were not. Status epilepticus also has a considerable morbidity, and is associated with the development of learning difficulties, focal neurological deficits and chronic epilepsy (Shorvon, 1994). Thus, the necessity of differentiating status from other seizure types is not solely phenomenological, but importantly relates to the high morbidity and mortality characterized by this condition.

Of all the forms of status epilepticus, convulsive status epilepticus carries the highest morbidity and mortality; it is also the commonest type (although this may partly be due to the better reporting of a potentially fatal condition than of milder, less easily diagnosed conditions). This chapter will thus concentrate on the use of benzodiazepines in the treatment of convulsive status epilepticus, and will only briefly discuss the role of benzodiazepines in the treatment of non-convulsive forms of status epilepticus.

STATUS EPILEPTICUS AS A STAGED CONDITION

Despite Gastaut's definition, status epilepticus is a varying condition and can be staged by physiological compromise, electrographic stages, occurrence of excitotoxicity, and responses to treatment. The poor prognosis of convulsive status epilepticus is largely due to the severe physiological compromise that occurs in the condition. The systemic effects of convulsive status epilepticus can be divided into early and late stages. The initial consequence of a prolonged convulsion is a massive release of plasma catecholamines (Benowitz et al., 1986), which results in an increase in heart rate, blood pressure and plasma glucose (Posner et al., 1968; Meldrum and Horton, 1973; Meldrum et al., 1979). Cerebral blood flow is greatly increased and thus glucose delivery to active cerebral tissue is maintained (Posner et al., 1968; Ingvar and Siesjö, 1983). This initial phase can be seen as a compensatory phase. As the seizure continues, there is a steady rise in the core body temperature, and acidosis, and cardiac arrhythmias also commonly occur (Aminoff and Simon, 1980).

The status epilepticus then enters a second phase, usually after a period of 60–90 minutes of seizure activity. The main characteristics of this phase are: a fall in blood pressure; a loss of cerebral autoregulation resulting in the dependence of cerebral blood flow on systemic blood pressure; and hypoglycaemia due to neurogenic insulin secretion and the exhaustion of glycogen stores (Meldrum and Horton, 1973; Wasterlain, 1974; Meldrum et al., 1979; Benowitz et al., 1986). This is the phase of decompensation. If this severe physiological compromise is not countered then it can result in both neuronal damage and widespread organ failure. It is thus imperative that patients at this stage are treated on an intensive care unit.

Neuronal damage also occurs that is independent of the physiological compromise. Critical animal experiments in the 1970s and 1980s demonstrated that even without the systemic disturbance associated with status epilepticus, neuronal damage still occurs (Meldrum, 1991). This neuronal damage is solely dependent upon the presence of electrographic seizure activity, and has been termed 'excitotoxicity'. In both animal models and humans, the degree of excitotoxic neuronal damage relates to the length of time of electrographic status epilepticus (Meldrum and Brierley, 1973; Sloviter, 1983; Nevander et al., 1985). Thus, as well as the physiological stages, status epilepticus can be staged according to the degree of excitotoxic neuronal damage.

Convulsive status epilepticus can also be temporally divided clinically and electrographically (Treiman, 1993; Shorvon, 1994). The initial stage is that of discrete seizures; then there is waxing and waning of ictal discharges, which progress to continuous ictal discharges. The final stages are continuous ictal discharges punctuated by flat periods, and then periodic epileptiform discharges on a flat background. The importance of these stages is that they not only relate to the underlying neuronal damage, but also to progressive difficulty in treating the status epilepticus (Table 1). The stage at which treatment is most effective is the first stage, which represents a premonitory phase

Table 1. Response of status epilepticus rat model to diazepam at different stages.

EEG group	No. of rats responding to 20 mg/kg diazepam
Discrete seizure	6/6
Waxing and waning	3/6
Continuous	1/6
PED	1/6

EEG, electroencephalogram; PED, periodic epileptiform discharges.
Source: Walton and Treiman (1988).

of progressively more frequent seizures. This stage is frequently encountered clinically and effective treatment usually prevents the development of 'true' status epilepticus.

This electroclinical progression, the advent of status-induced neuronal damage and the physiological effects described above have resulted in the development of temporal regimens in the drug treatment of convulsive status epilepticus. There are three main treatment stages: the premonitory stage; the stage of established status epilepticus; and the stage of refractory status epilepticus (Shorvon, 1994).

THE USE OF BENZODIAZEPINES IN STATUS EPILEPTICUS

Convulsive status epilepticus is, for the reasons outlined above, a medical emergency, and requires prompt, effective treatment. Because of benzo-diazepines' rapid onset of action and efficacy against seizures, they seem ideal drugs for the treatment of status epilepticus. Indeed, soon after diazepam's first clinical use, its potency in treating status epilepticus was realized (Gastaut *et al.*, 1965) and it has now become one of the first-line treatments for this condition (Shorvon, 1994). Since then, four benzo-diazepines have predominantly been used in convulsive status epilepticus: diazepam, lorazepam, midazolam and clonazepam.

Benzodiazepines are effective at all stages of status epilepticus in humans and animal models, and are amongst the most successful drugs used for this condi-tion. Although their primary mode of action is to enhance gamma-aminobutyric acid (GABA)ergic inhibition via the benzodiazepine receptor (Macdonald, 1989), other modes of action probably contribute at the doses used in status epilepticus. Indeed, clonazepam, lorazepam and diazepam, at concentrations similar to that necessary to halt status epilepticus, can reduce rapid repetitive firing in a similar fashion to carbamazepine and phenytoin – drugs that act at voltage-dependent sodium channels (McLean and Macdonald, 1988).

The effectiveness of benzodiazepines decreases as status epilepticus progresses (Table 1), so that at the stage of 'discrete seizures' in a pilocarpine/lithium rat model of status epilepticus, 20 mg/kg diazepam stops seizures in 100% of the rats tested, but by the stage of 'periodic discharges', the same dose is effective in only 17% of the rats (Walton and Treiman, 1988). Similarly, studies in pilocarpine-induced status epilepticus demon-strate that the ED_{50} of diazepam increases by a factor of 10 from 10 minutes of seizure activity to 45 minutes of seizure activity (Kapur and Macdonald, 1997). Importantly, this represents a decrease in potency rather than efficacy of diazepam. On a cellular level, this decrease in potency is associated with a decrease in the sensitivity of GABA receptors to diazepam (Kapur and Macdonald, 1997).

PHARMACOKINETICS OF ACUTELY ADMINISTERED
BENZODIAZEPINES

Drugs used in status epilepticus need to have a rapid onset of action. In order to accomplish this, the drugs need to cross the blood–brain barrier readily. Antiepileptic drugs achieve this either by being lipid soluble or by having an active transport mechanism (Loscher and Frey, 1984). This has led to many drugs that are effective in status epilepticus having a high lipid solubility, and thus a large volume of distribution and a biphasic concentration versus time curve (Figure 1).

Benzodiazepines are no exception to this, and their acute pharmacokinetics are predominantly determined by redistribution into peripheral compartments. Within the benzodiazepines, however, there is a large variability in pharmacokinetic profiles.

Diazepam is the most widely used benzodiazepine in status epilepticus. It has a redistribution half-life of less than 1 hour with a large volume of distribution of 1–2 l/kg, and an elimination half-life of 20–40 hours. Because of its high lipophilicity, it rapidly crosses the blood–brain barrier resulting in a fast onset of action (Greenblatt et al., 1980; Arendt et al., 1983; Friedman, et al., 1986; Schmidt, 1995). Given as an intravenous bolus, it halts status epilepticus in approximately 80% of patients in a matter of minutes (Schmidt, 1995). The short distribution half-life, however, results in a rapid fall in serum concentration and a concomitant fall in brain concentration, leading to recurrence of seizure activity (Greenblatt and Sethy, 1990; Schmidt, 1995). Within 2 hours of successful treatment with diazepam, over half the patients with status epilepticus relapse (Prensky et al., 1967). For this reason, repeat intravenous boluses or a continuous infusion of diazepam are commonly used. Repeat doses of diazepam, however, lead to significant decrease in volume

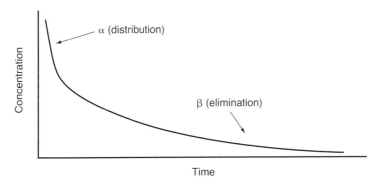

Figure 1. Acute pharmacokinetics of lipid-soluble drugs often are biphasic with a rapid distribution phase followed by a slower elimination phase.

of distribution, and a decrease in clearance leading to greater peak concentrations and relative persistence (Walker *et al.*, 1998). Furthermore, the (CSF) levels of diazepam following repeat dosing are maintained for longer than would be predicted from the serum data probably due to accumulation within the brain from non-specific binding (Walker *et al.*, 1998). Thus, although the blood concentrations drop precipitously following a single bolus as a result of redistribution, infusions and repeat boluses lead to accumulation and therefore to persistent action (Walker *et al.*, 1998). This can result in sudden hypotension, and respiratory and circulatory collapse.

Clonazepam shares many of the pharmacokinetic features of diazepam. It has a similarly rapid brain penetration, short distribution half-life and long elimination half-life (Pinder *et al.*, 1976; Greenblatt et al., 1987). Lorazepam, on the other hand, has a smaller volume distribution and is less lipid soluble. It enters the brain more slowly, taking up to 30 minutes to achieve peak brain levels (Greenblatt *et al.*, 1989). This corresponds to its peak pharmacodynamic effect (Greenblatt *et al.*, 1989). Its distribution half-life is much longer, 2–3 hours, and its elimination half-life is shorter, approximately 10–12 hours (Greenblatt *et al.*, 1989). These characteristics result in a slower onset of action, but a longer duration of action. Lorazepam and clonazepam have a much greater affinity for the benzodiazepine receptor compared with diazepam; it has been suggested that lorazepam's longer duration of action is due to its decreased rate of receptor dissociation. Although this is an appealing hypothesis, more recent evidence suggests that the duration of action of these three drugs can be explained solely by their pharmacokinetics (Greenblatt and Sethy, 1990).

Midazolam's use in status epilepticus is more recent. Midazolam has a very short distribution half-life of less than 5 minutes, and a very short elimination half-life of approximately 1.5 hours (Bell *et al.*, 1991). These characteristics and its smaller volume of distribution make it the benzodiazepine of choice for use as an infusion because it has less propensity to accumulate.

USE OF BENZODIAZEPINES AT DIFFERENT STAGES OF STATUS EPILEPTICUS

Premonitory stage

This is the stage of increasingly frequent seizures that occurs prior to hospitalization. Thus, what is needed is a drug that can be given by a route that can be used outside the hospital setting, yet still has a rapid onset of action, and should not be complicated by respiratory or circulatory problems. Rectal diazepam has generally been the drug of choice (Shorvon, 1994). Neither suppositories nor oral diazepam has a fast enough onset of action, and intramuscular diazepam has the problem of local irritation and erratic absorption. A solution of 0.5–1 mg/kg rectal diazepam results in therapeutic serum concentrations within 1 hour, and has been shown to be very effective in arresting acute seizures with minimal side effects (Dreifuss *et al.*, 1998).

A possible disadvantage of rectal diazepam is concern about and difficulties in the route of administration, especially in children; alternatives have therefore been sought. Midazolam has the advantage over other benzodiazepines of being water soluble at a suitable pH; at physiological pH it becomes highly lipophilic, permitting rapid transfer across the blood–brain barrier. This has resulted in the possibility of midazolam usage by three other routes: intranasal, buccal and intramuscular (Bell *et al.*, 1991; Rey *et al.*, 1991; Scott *et al.*, 1998). Of these, the buccal modazolam seems to be the most promising: it is as effective as rectal diazepam in acute seizures, and is easy to administer (Scott *et al.*, 1999). By this route, the maximum concentration is reached by 30 minutes (although the pharmacodynamic response may be quicker), and the bioavailability is 75%. Intranasal midazolam has also been used successfully: a dose of 0.2 mg/kg intranasally results in a maximum serum concentration in 12 minutes with a bioavailability of 55% (Rey *et al.*, 1991).

Established status epilepticus (30–60 minutes)

At this stage intravenous medication is needed. The ideal treatment should be efficacious, fast acting, should have a persistent action, and should not cause respiratory or circulatory problems. Diazepam has been the drug of choice, but its short distribution half-life has meant that it is usually given with a longer-acting drug such as phenytoin, and is often used as repeat boluses (Delgado Escueta and Enrile Bacsal, 1983). It is, however, very effective. Clonazepam appears to offer little advantage over diazepam. Lorazepam, however, has a longer duration of action, but a slower rate of brain penetration. Lorazepam and diazepam have been compared in a randomized study in which both were equally effective – seizure cessation resulted in 89% and 76% respectively (Leppik *et al.*, 1983). In a recent multi-centre, double-blind, randomized study of initial treatment of status epilepticus, there was no statistical difference between the efficacy of lorazepam 0.1 mg/kg and the combination of diazepam 0.15 mg/kg and phenytoin 18 mg/kg (Treiman *et al.*, 1998). Lorazepam was, however, easier to use and was faster to administer. There was also no difference in side effects (Treiman *et al.*, 1998). One criticism of this comparison is that the dose of diazepam that was used is lower than that usually used in the UK of 0.2–0.3 mg/kg. Although there is little evidence supporting one benzodiazepine over another at this stage, lorazepam probably has the advantages of a longer duration of action and ease of administration.

Refractory status epilepticus (60–90 minutes)

At this stage the physiological compromise and the dangers of further drug treatment mean that transfer to the intensive care unit is mandatory (Walker *et al.*, 1995). It is important to abolish electrographic seizure activity as quickly as possible to prevent excitotoxicity, and thus induction of general anaesthesia is the preferred treatment (Walker *et al.*, 1995). The agents that are commonly used are barbiturate anaesthetics (thiopentone or pentobarbital), propofol and midazolam. Midazolam is the benzodiazepine of choice at this stage because it has a lesser propensity to accumulate, and a shorter half-life enabling easier and more rapid control of the degree of anaesthesia. It has been successfully used in both children and adults at a dose of approximately 0.15 mg/kg followed by an infusion of 0.05–0.4 mg/kg per hour (Kumar and Bleck, 1992; Rivera *et al.*, 1993; Parent and Lowenstein, 1994; Sheth *et al.*, 1996; Lal Koul *et al.*, 1997). In the intensive care setting it is worth noting that midazolam can have a greater half-life and volume of distribution, and that prolonged infusions can result in accumulation (Malacrida *et al.*, 1992). The dose should be titrated against electrographic seizure suppression using an electroencephalogram (EEG) or cerebral function monitor. Whether an EEG burst suppression pattern or an isoelectric EEG is preferable to just seizure suppression is unknown, but both these electrographic targets require much higher doses of anaesthetic with a consequent increased risk of side effects (Walker *et al.*, 1996). Following 24 hours of seizure suppression, the anaesthetic should be slowly tapered providing that there are adequate doses of other antiepileptic drugs present.

NON-CONVULSIVE STATUS EPILEPTICUS

The two main forms of non-convulsive status epilepticus are complex partial status epilepticus and absence status epilepticus; in both of these, benzodiazepines form the mainstay of treatment.

Complex partial status epilepticus

The correct diagnosis of complex partial status presents one of the major difficulties with this condition. Not only does it have to be differentiated from other forms of non-convulsive status epilepticus, but also from post-ictal states and other neurological and psychiatric conditions. EEG may be helpful, but often the scalp EEG changes are non-specific and the diagnosis is very much clinical in nature (Cascino, 1993; Shorvon, 1994). Shorvon (1994) defined complex partial status epilepticus as 'a prolonged epileptic episode in which focal fluctuating or frequently recurring electrographic epileptic discharges, arising in temporal or extratemporal regions, result in a confusional state with variable clinical symptoms'.

How aggressively complex partial status epilepticus is treated depends upon: (1) the prognosis of the condition; (2) whether treatment improves the prognosis. As in all epilepsies, the prognosis relates to the prognosis of the underlying aetiology and any concomitant medical conditions. Animal models of limbic (complex partial) status result in neuronal damage similar to that seen in convulsive status. Human data, however, are less compelling. There have been reports of prolonged memory problems, hemiparesis and death occurring following complex partial status epilepticus, although in many of these cases, the outcome relates to the underlying cause (Treiman *et al.*, 1981; Cascino, 1993; Krumholz *et al.*, 1995). Furthermore, in many of these cases the complex partial status epilepticus is treated aggressively with barbiturate anaesthesia, and the treatment itself could have resulted in the morbidity observed. In addition, there have been reports of prolonged complex partial status epilepticus with no neurological sequelae (Williamson *et al.*, 1985; Cockerell *et al.*, 1994). A recent study of eight patients demonstrated that despite the absence of an acute neurological insult, complex partial status epilepticus resulted in significant rises in serum neuron-specific enolase, a marker for acute neuronal injury (DeGiorgio *et al.*, 1996). In this study, there was no correlation between duration of seizure and the serum neuron-specific enolase, although this may be the result of the small sample size because larger studies in status epilepticus have found such a correlation (DeGiorgio *et al.*, 1995). The degree to which serum neuronal-specific enolase correlates with neurological and cognitive disability in complex partial status epilepticus, and whether the results of this pilot study are true for the majority of patients (especially those with recurrent complex partial status epilepticus) are unknown. Early recognition is paramount.

Treatment should begin with oral or rectal benzodiazepines, and oral clobazam is possibly the benzodiazepine of choice (Corman *et al.*, 1998). For more persistent complex partial status epilepticus, intravenous therapy, as with convulsive status epilepticus, should be used, but whether general anaesthesia is justified remains a matter for speculation; since most complex partial status epilepticus is self-terminating, often without any serious neurological sequelae (Cockerell *et al.*, 1994), then such aggressive therapy should perhaps be avoided.

ABSENCE STATUS EPILEPTICUS

This entity needs to be distinguished from complex partial status epilepticus and atypical absences seen in mental retardation (Cascino, 1993; Shorvon, 1994).

This term should perhaps be reserved for prolonged absence attacks with continuous or discontinuous 3 Hz spike and wave occurring in patients with primary generalized epilepsy (Cockerell *et al.*, 1994; Shorvon, 1994). The EEG, however, may include irregular spike/wave, prolonged bursts of spike activity, and sharp wave or polyspike and wave, and whether to include such cases as absence status epilepticus is uncertain (Shorvon, 1994; Porter and Penry, 1983). Conversely, there can be runs of 3-Hz spike and wave during complex partial status epilepticus.

Although absence epilepsy has its peak in childhood and commonly remits in adolescence, absence status epilepticus commonly occurs in later life. Absence status epilepticus can be divided into childhood absence status epilepticus (those usually already receiving treatment), late-onset absence status epilepticus with a history of primary generalized history (often a history of absences in childhood) and late-onset absence status epilepticus developing *de novo* (usually following drug, often benzodiazepine, or alcohol withdrawal) (Shorvon, 1994).

There is no evidence that absence status induces neuronal damage, and thus aggressive treatment is rarely warranted (Porter and Penry, 1983; Shorvon, 1994). Treatment can either be intravenous or oral. Absence status epilepticus responds very rapidly to intravenous benzodiazepines, and these are so effective that the response is both diagnostic and therapeutic.

CONCLUSION

Benzodiazepines are the most efficacious and potent drugs available for the treatment of status epilepticus, and form an integral part of any protocol. The authors' favoured protocol for the treatment of convulsive status epilepticus is contained in Table 2. The choice of benzodiazepines at each stage of

Table 2. Authors' proposed protocol for the treatment of convulsive status epilepticus in adults.

Stage	Authors' preference	Alternatives
Premonitory	Rectal diazepam 10–20 mg	Buccal, intramuscular or intranasal midazolam
Initial	Lorazepam 4 mg, repeat after 10 min	Diazepam 20 mg, repeat after 10 min
Then	Phenytoin 15–18 mg/kg at 50 mg/min	Phenobarbitone 10–20 mg/kg at 100 mg/min
Late (anaesthesia)	Propofol 2 mg/kg then 5–10 mg/kg per hour	Midazolam 5–10 mg then 0.05–0.4 mg/kg per hour Thiopentone 100–250 mg then 3–5 mg/kg per hour Pentobarbitone 5–20 mg/kg then 0.5–3 mg/kg per hour

status epilepticus is mainly determined by their pharmacokinetic and physio-chemical properties.

REFERENCES

Aminoff, M.J. and Simon R.P. (1980). Status epilepticus: causes, clinical features and consequences in 98 patients. *Am J Med* **69**, 657–666.

Arendt, R.M., Greenblatt, D.J., deJong, R.H. *et al.* (1983). In vitro correlates of benzodiazepine cerebrospinal fluid uptake, pharmacodynamic action and peripheral distribution. *J Pharmacol Exp Ther* **227**, 95–106.

Bell, D.M., Richards, G., Dhillon, S. *et al.* (1991). A comparative pharmacokinetic study of intravenous and intramuscular midazolam in patients with epilepsy. *Epilepsy Res* **10**(2–3), 183–190.

Benowitz, N.L., Simon, R.P. and Copeland, J.R. (1986). Status epilepticus: divergence of sympathetic activity and cardiovascular response. *Ann Neurol* **19**, 197–199.

Calmeil, J.-L. (1824). De l'épilepsie, étudiée sous le rapport de son siège et de son influence sur la production de l'aliénation mentale. Thesis, Université de Paris.

Cascino, G.D. (1993). Nonconvulsive status epilepticus in adults and children. *Epilepsia* **34**, S21–S28.

Cockerell, O.C., Walker, M.C., Sander, J.W. and Shorvon, S.D. (1994). Complex partial status epilepticus: a recurrent problem. *J Neurol Neurosurg Psychiatry* **57**, 835–837.

Corman, C., Guberman, A. and Benavente, O. (1998). Clobazam in partial status epilepticus. *Seizure* **7**, 243–247.

DiGiorgio, C.M., Correale, J.D., Gott, P.S. *et al.* (1995). Serum neuron-specific enolase in human status epilepticus. *Neurology* **45**, 1134–1137.

DiGiorgio, C.M., Gott, P.S., Rabinowicz, A.L., Heck, C.N., Smith, T. and Correale, J.D. (1996). Neuron-specific enolase, a marker of acute neuronal injury, is increased in complex partial status epilepticus. *Epilepsia* **36**, 475–479.

Delgado-Escueta, A.V. and Enrile Bacsal, F. (1983). Combination therapy for status epilepticus: intravenous diazepam and phenytoin. *Adv Neurol* **34**, 477–485.

DeLorenzo, R.J., Hauser, W.A., Towne, A.R. *et al.* (1996). A prospective, population-based epidemiologic study of status epilepticus in Richmond, Virginia. (1993). *Neurology* **46**(4), 1029–1035.

Dreifuss, F.E., Rosman, N.P., Cloyd, J.C. *et al.* (1998). A comparison of rectal diazepam gel and placebo for acute repetitive seizures. *N Engl J Med* **338**, 1869–1875.

Friedman, H., Abernethy, D.R., Greenblatt, D.J. and Shader, R.I. (1986). The pharmacokinetics of diazepam and desmethyldiazepam in rat brain and plasma. *Psychopharmacology* **88**, 267–270.

Gastaut, H. (1973). *Dictionary of Epilepsy. Part 1 Definitions.* Geneva: World Health Organization.

Gastaut, H., Naquet, R., Poire, R. and Tassinari, C.A. (1965). Treatment of status epilepticus with diazepam (valium). *Epilepsia* **6**, 167–182.

Gastaut, H., Roger, J. and Lob, H. (1967). *Les États de Mal Épileptiques.* Masson, Paris.

Greenblatt, D.J. and Sethy, V.H. (1990). Benzodiazepine concentrations in brain directly reflect receptor occupancy: studies of diazepam and oxazepam. *Psychopharmacology* **102**, 373–378.

Greenblatt, D.J., Ochs, H.R. and Lloyd, B.L. (1980). Entry of diazepam and its major metabolite into cerebrospinal fluid. *Psychopharmacology* **70**, 89–93.

Greenblatt, D.J., Miller, L.G. and Shader, R.I. (1987). Clonazepam pharmacokinetics, brain uptake, and receptor interactions. *J Clin Psychiatry* **48**(suppl), 4–11.

Greenblatt, D.J., Ehrenberg, B.L., Gunderman, J. *et al.* (1989). Kinetic and dynamic study of intravenous lorazepam: comparison with intravenous diazepam. *J Pharmacol Exp Ther* **250**(1), 134–140.

Ingvar, M.H. and Siesjö, B.K. (1983). Local blood flow glucose consumption in the rat brain during sustained bicuculline-induced seizures. *Acta Neurol Scand* **68**, 128–144.

Kapur, J. and Macdonald, R.L. (1997). Rapid seizure-related reduction of benzodiazepine and Zn2+ sensitivity of hippocampal dentate granule cell GABAA receptors. *J Neurosci* **17**(19), 7532–7540.

Krumholz, A., Sung, G.Y., Fisher, R.S., Barry, E., Bergey, G.K. and Gratten, L.M. (1995). Complex partial status epilepticus accompanied by serious morbidity and mortality. *Neurology* **45**, 1499–1504.

Kumar, A. and Bleck, T.P. (1992). Intravenous midazolam for the treatment of refractory status epilepticus. *Crit Care Med* **20**, 483–488.

Lal Koul, R., Raj Aithala, G., Chacko, A., Joshi, R. and Serif Elbualy, M. (1997). Continuous midazolam infusion as treatment of status epilepticus. *Arch Dis Child* **76**, 445–448.

Leppik, I.E., Derivan, A.T., Homan, R.W., Walker, J., Ramsay, R.E. and Patrick, B. (1983). Double-blind study of lorazepam and diazepam in status epilepticus. *JAMA* **249**, 1452–1454.

Loscher, W. and Frey, H.-H. (1984). Kinetics of penetration of common antiepileptic drugs into cerebrospinal fluid. *Epilepsia* **25**, 346–352.

Lowenstein, D.H., Bleck, T. and Macdonald, R.L. (1999). It's time to revise the definition of status epilepticus. *Epilepsia* **40**, 120–122.

Macdonald, R.L. (1989). Antiepileptic drug actions. *Epilepsia* **30**(suppl 1), S19–S28.

Malacrida, R., Fritz, M.E., Suter, P.M. and Crevoisier, C. (1992). Pharmacokinetics of midazolam administered by continuous intravenous infusion to intensive care patients. *Crit Care Med* **20**, 1123–1126.

McLean, M.J. and Macdonald, R.L. (1988). Benzodiazepines, but not beta carbolines, limit high frequency repetitive firing of action potentials of spinal cord neurons in cell culture. *J Pharmacol Exp Ther* **244**, 789–795.

Meldrum, B. (1991). Excitotoxicity and epileptic brain damage. *Epilepsy Res* **10**, 55–61.

Meldrum, B.S. and Brierley, J.B. (1973). Prolonged epileptic seizures in primates. Ischaemic cell change and its relation to ictal physiological events. *Arch Neurol* **28**, 10–17.

Meldrum, B.S. and Horton, R.W. (1973). Physiology of status epilepticus in primates. *Arch Neurol* **28**, 1–9.

Meldrum, B.S., Horton, R.W., Blood, S.R., Butler, J. and Keenan, J. (1979). Endocrine factors in glucose metabolism during prolonged seizures in baboons. *Epilepsia* **20**, 527–534.

Nevander, G., Ingvar, M., Auer, A. and Siesjö, B.K. (1985). Status epilepticus in well-oxygenated rats causes neuronal necrosis. *Ann Neurol* **18**, 281–290.

Parent, J.M. and Lowenstein, D.H. (1994). Treatment of refractory generalized status epilepticus with continuous infusion of midazolam. *Neurology* **44**, 1837–1840.

Pinder, R.M., Brogden, R.N., Speight, T.M. and Avery, G.S. (1976). Clonazepam: a review of its pharmacological properties and therapeutic efficacy in epilepsy. *Drugs* **12**, 321–361.

Porter, R.J. and Penry, J.K. (1983). Petit mal status. *Adv Neurol* **34**, 61–67.

Posner, J.B., Plum, F. and Troy, B. (1968). Cerebral metabolic and circulatory responses to induced convulsions in animals. *Arch Neurol* **18**, 1–13.

Prensky, A.L., Raff, M.C., Moore, M.J. and Schwab, R.S. (1967). Intravenous diazepam in the treatment of prolonged seizure activity. *N Engl J Med* **276**, 779–784.

Rey, E., Delaunay, L., Pons, G. *et al.* (1991). Pharmacokinetics of midazolam in children: comparative study of intranasal and intravenous administration. *Eur J Clin Pharmacol* **41**, 355–357.

Rivera, R., Segnini, M., Baltodano, A. and Perez, V. (1993). Midazolam in the treatment of status epilepticus in children. *Crit Care Med* **21**, 991–994.

Schmidt, D. (1995). Diazepam. In: Levy, R.H., Mattson, R.H. and Meldrum, B.S. (Eds), *Antiepileptic Drugs*. Raven Press, New York, pp. 705–724.

Scott, R.C., Besag, F.M., Boyd, S.G., Berry, D. and Neville, B.G. (1998). Buccal absorption of midazolam: pharmacokinetics and EEG pharmacodynamics. *Epilepsia* **39**(3), 290–294.

Scott, R.C., Besag, F.M. and Neville, B.G. (1999). Buccal midazolam and rectal diazepam for treatment of prolonged seizures in childhood and adolescence: a randomised trial. *Lancet* **353**, 623–626.

Sheth, R.D., Buckley, D.J., Gutierrez, A.R., Gingold, M., Bodensteiner, J.B. and Penney, S. (1996). Midazolam in the treatment of refractory neonatal seizures. *Clin Neuropharmacol* **19**, 165–170.

Shorvon, S.D. (1994). *Status Epilepticus: its Clinical Features and Treatment in Children and Adults*. Cambridge University Press, Cambridge.

Sloviter, R.S. (1983). 'Epileptic' brain damage in rats induced by sustained electrical stimulation of the perforant path, I. Acute electrophysiological and light microscopic studies. *Brain Res Bull* **10**, 675–697.

Treiman, D.M. (1993). Generalised convulsive status epilepticus in the adult. *Epilepsia* **34**, S2–S11.

Treiman, D.M., Delgado-Escueta, A.V. and Clark, M.A. (1981). Impairment of memory following prolonged complex partial status epilepticus. *Neurology* **31**, 109.

Treiman, D.M., Meyers, P.D., Walton, N.Y. *et al.* (1998). A comparison of four treatments for generalized convulsive status epilepticus. Veterans Affairs Status Epilepticus Cooperative Study Group. *N Engl J Med* **339**, 792–798.

Walker, M.C., Smith, S.J. and Shorvon, S.D. (1995). The intensive care treatment of convulsive status epilepticus in the UK. Results of a national survey and recommendations. *Anaesthesia* **50**, 130–135.

Walker, M.C., Howard, R.S., Smith, S.J., Miller, D.H., Shorvon, S.D. and Hirsch, N.P. (1996). Diagnosis and treatment of status epilepticus on a neurological intensive care unit. *QJM* **89**, 913–920.

Walker, M.C., Tong, X., Brown, S., Shorvon, S.D. and Patsalos, P.N. (1998). Comparison of single- and repeated-dose pharmacokinetics of diazepam. *Epilepsia* **39**, 283–289.

Walton, N.Y. and Treiman, D.M. (1988). Response of status epileptics induced by lithium and pilocarpine to treatment with diazepam. *Exp Neurol* **101**, 267–275.

Wasterlain, C.G. (1974). Mortality and morbidity from serial seizures. An experimental study. *Epilepsia* **15**, 155–176.

Williamson, P.D., Spencer, D.D., Spencer, S.S., Novelly, R.A. and Mattson, R.H. (1985). Complex partial status epilepticus: a depth-electrode study. *Ann Neurol* **18**, 647–654.

Benzodiazepines
Edited by Michael R. Trimble and Ian Hindmarch
© 2000 Wrightson Biomedical Publishing Ltd

8

The Use of Benzodiazepines in Childhood Epilepsy

JOHN H. LIVINGSTON

Department of Paediatric Neurology, Leeds General Infirmary, Leeds, UK

INTRODUCTION

Benzodiazepines have become widely used in the treatment of severe childhood epilepsy since their introduction four decades ago. At that time there was a relatively small number of antiepileptic drugs (AED) to choose from. The availability of benzodiazepines was thus a breakthrough. Since then, however, many more AEDs are available and the role of the benzodiazepines has become more limited. This chapter will consider the current role of benzodiazepines in the management of childhood epilepsy.

GENERAL CONSIDERATIONS

Benzodiazepines are extremely potent AEDs with efficacy against a wide spectrum of seizure types (Ko *et al.*, 1997; Schmidt, 1985). Three major problems, however, limit their use as oral AEDs in childhood. First, compared with other AEDs they have a high rate of behavioural and cognitive effects (Schmidt, 1985; Bourgeois, 1996; Ko *et al.*, 1997). In children, this may manifest either as cognitive slowing, which may be quite severe, or as marked behavioural changes, often with agitation, aggression and over-activity, and occasionally quite severe psychomotor regression. These effects are often so marked that even if there has been a significant improvement in seizure control, the carers will opt to discontinue treatment. In addition to the behavioural and cognitive effects, benzodiazepines may cause hypotonia, ataxia, drooling and excessive bronchial secretions.

Table 1. Recommended doses for starting and stopping benzodiazepines.

	Starting dose (mg/kg per day)	Max. dose (mg/kg per day)	No. of daily doses	Rate of withdrawal
Nitrazepam	0.05	0.5–1	2–3	0.25 mg/day every 2 weeks
Clonazepam	0.01–0.03	0.2–0.3	2–3	0.125 mg/day every 2 weeks
Clobazam	0.25	1	2	2.5 mg/day every 2 weeks

Secondly, withdrawal seizures, including status epilepticus, occur very frequently on attempted discontinuation especially if this is done abruptly (Lund and Trolle, 1973; Allen *et al.*, 1983; Schmidt, 1985). Withdrawal seizures are more likely when there has been chronic administration for several months or longer. If the patient has developed tolerance (see below) then there is the difficult predicament of continuing on an ineffective AED, which may be having adverse effects but which leads to withdrawal seizures on attempted dose reduction. If these patients or their parents/carers have had bad experiences with withdrawal seizures they may be very reluctant to reconsider dose reduction. This in turn may lead to polytherapy with its associated problems. For these reasons, withdrawal of benzodiazepines in those who have been on chronic treatment needs to be carried out very carefully (Table 1).

Thirdly, tolerance to the antiepileptic effects develops in a high proportion of children. Tolerance has been variously defined. Usually the term refers to a deterioration of seizure control in a patient with previously good control, in whom increasing the dose does not result in an improvement (Haigh and Feely 1988). Tolerance has been reported to occur in up to 86% of patients within 3–12 months of starting therapy (Robertson, 1986; Schmidt *et al.*, 1986a). Increasing the dose usually has no effect on seizure control but often increases adverse effects.

Tolerance is a problem with all of the benzodiazepines, and cross-tolerance often, but not always, occurs (Schmidt *et al.*, 1986a; Schoch *et al.*, 1993). The mechanism of tolerance is not fully understood (see Chapter 9).

These significant problems mean that oral benzodiazepines are not usually considered as first line treatment in any childhood epilepsies. The overall role has been as third- or fourth-line AEDs in severe childhood epilepsy syndromes or in other epilepsies that have been resistant to first- or second-line AEDs.

SPECIFIC BENZODIAZEPINES

The oral benzodiazepines that have been most widely used in children are, in order of their historical development:

- nitrazepam
- clonazepam
- clobazam.

See Table 1 for recommended doses.

Nitrazepam

Nitrazepam has been used in the treatment of childhood epilepsy since 1963. Nitrazepam is a 1,4-benzodiazepine that is usually given orally. It is absorbed completely and is lipophilic, crossing membranes readily. The elimination half-life is long and the drug accumulates with daily use (Reider and Wendt, 1973). Nitrazepam is metabolized in the liver; the metabolites are inactive and are excreted in the urine.

Nitrazepam has been found to be useful against various childhood seizures and epilepsies with efficacy against infantile spasms, myoclonic seizures, atypical absences, generalized tonic clonic seizures, partial seizures and Lennox–Gastaut syndrome (Browne and Penry, 1973; Schmidt, 1985; Ko *et al.*, 1997).

Largely for historical reasons, nitrazepam has become particularly associated with the treatment of infantile spasms (Carson, 1968; Schmidt, 1983; Burdette and Browne, 1990).

Comparative studies of the use of nitrazepam versus steroids in infantile spasms have demonstrated similar efficacy (Dreifuss *et al.*, 1986). The number of patients experiencing adverse effects was also similar although the steroid group had more severe side effects.

Many of the early reports on the use of nitrazepam demonstrated efficacy against myoclonic seizures, particularly in infants (Liske and Forster, 1963; Millichap and Ortiz, 1966). For many years nitrazepam was widely used to treat myoclonic and other seizures in infants with evolving cerebral palsy. This was often associated with a high rate of adverse effects, particularly sedation, behavioural change and excess bronchial secretions. No comparative studies with other AEDs in this group of patients have been performed. It is likely that other AEDs are as effective but better tolerated in these patients and nitrazepam now would be seen as a third- or fourth-line agent.

Clonazepam

Clonazepam is a chlorinated derivative of nitrazepam that has been widely used as an adjunctive treatment in childhood epilepsy. The absorption of oral clonazepam is 80% or more and peak levels occur within 1–4 hours of oral administration. Distribution is rapid and clonazepam is metabolized by nitro reduction and acetylation. Neither metabolite appears to have pharmacological activity. Elimination of clonazepam is slow, with a half-life of 20–80 hours (Dreifuss *et al.*, 1975; Andre *et al.*, 1991). Clonazepam is available as a liquid, in tablet form and as an intravenous preparation.

Clonazepam has efficacy against many childhood seizure types, both partial and generalized (Ishikawa *et al.*, 1985). Reports in children mainly concern severe and intractable epilepsy syndromes (Browne, 1976; Farrell, 1986). Clonazepam has some efficacy against infantile spasms but seems less effective than adrenocorticotropic hormone (Vasella *et al.*, 1973; Browne, 1976). Although no comparative studies have been published, nitrazepam does seem more effective in infantile spasms than clonazepam.

Clonazepam has been widely used in Lennox–Gastaut syndrome and has efficacy against tonic clonic, atypical absence, tonic, myoclonic and atonic seizures (Vasella *et al.*, 1973; O'Donohoe and Paes, 1977; Schmidt, 1985).

Adverse effects are common. The most common being drowsiness, behavioural change and ataxia (Browne, 1983). Other adverse effects include hypotonia, dysarthria and excessive bronchial secretions (Burdette and Browne, 1990).

Clobazam

Clobazam is a 1,5-benzodiazepine that has been in clinical use as an AED since 1978 (Gastaut, 1978). It is available only as an oral preparation.

After oral administration clobazam is virtually completely absorbed. Peak levels occur within 1–3 hours. Clobazam is highly lipophilic and has a large volume of distribution. The half-life ranges from 10 to 55 hours (Ko *et al.*, 1997). It has been suggested that the antiepileptic activity of clobazam may be more attributable to *N*-desmethylclobazam than to clobazam itself (Meldrum and Croucher, 1982).

Clobazam has efficacy against a wide spectrum of seizure types including atypical absence, generalized tonic clonic seizures, myoclonic seizures and partial seizures (Allen *et al.*, 1983; Koeppen, 1985; Schmidt, 1994). There have been many reports documenting the efficacy of clobazam as add-on therapy in poorly controlled epilepsy (Koeppen, 1985; Keene *et al.*, 1990).

The most recent and largest study of the use of clobazam in childhood epilepsy was a prospective, randomized, comparative study of clobazam versus carbamazepine or phenytoin (Canadian Study Group for Childhood Epilepsy, 1998). Entry criteria for this study were age between 6 months to 17 years, epilepsy (defined as two or more unprovoked seizures) and a seizure type that was either partial or partial with secondary generalized or 'primary' generalized tonic clonic seizures. Patients with myoclonic, atonic, tonic or absence seizures were excluded. Patients either had newly diagnosed epilepsy or had experienced a previous failure of one AED for lack of efficacy or adverse effects.

A total of 235 children were entered into the study; 119 received clobazam, 78 carbamazepine and 38 phenytoin. Overall there was no difference in efficacy between all three drugs with 56% of patients still taking the original medication after 1 year. The incidence of adverse effects was similar for all three AEDs, although clobazam induced slightly more behavioural effects than carbamazepine or phenytoin (34% versus 29%).

Tolerance occurred in only 7.5% of patients receiving clobazam versus 4.2% and 6.7% for carbamazepine and phenytoin respectively. This study concluded that clobazam was equally effective as carbamazepine and phenytoin as monotherapy for newly diagnosed epilepsy.

Another way of expressing this result would be that clobazam was equally ineffective in these childhood epilepsies, with seizure control after 3 years of only 55%. This study has the limitations of all large multicentre studies of epilepsy particularly in relation to the ascertainment of the type of seizure or epilepsy syndrome. It does, however, demonstrate that clobazam may be well tolerated as monotherapy.

In this study, tolerance was quite strictly defined and occurred in only 7.5% of patients. This compares with a rate of 15–20% of patients developing tolerance in the Canadian retrospective study, which included both adults and children (Canadian Clobazam Co-operative Group, 1990). Both these studies had much lower rates of tolerance than previous studies, which suggested rates up to 86% (Singh et al., 1995). Comparing the reported rates of tolerance between studies is, however, difficult because different definitions have been used and different patient populations studied. This is discussed further in Chapter 9.

Overall, tolerance occurs in one third to one half of patients receiving clobazam for 1–6 months (Schmidt et al., 1986b; Remy, 1994). Side effects occur in at least 25% of patients receiving clobazam (Remy, 1994); these are mainly sedation, ataxia, memory problems and behavioural changes.

Clobazam has no significant interaction with other antiepileptic drugs, although it does lead to a decrease in the clearance of valproate and co-administration of phenobarbitone may decrease the clobazam level (Theis et al., 1997). Neither of these effects is likely to be of major clinical significance (Sheth et al., 1995).

There are few comparative studies of one benzodiazepine with another. Tolerance is a problem with all of them, but there is, however, an impression that adverse effects may be less with clobazam than with clonazepam or nitrazepam (Schmidt, 1985; Ko et al., 1997). Cross-tolerance generally, but not always, occurs and occasionally children will have a good response to one benzodiazepine having not responded or become tolerant to another. There is no justification for using two different benzodiazepines together.

BENZODIAZEPINES IN CHILDHOOD EPILEPSY

The role of benzodiazepines in the following epilepsies will now be considered:

- infantile spasms
- Lennox–Gastaut syndrome and other epileptic encephalopathies
- other epilepsy syndromes.

Infantile spasms

Infantile spasms refers to an epilepsy syndrome characterized by the occurrence of epileptic spasms in infancy and an abnormal interictal electroencephalogram. Infantile spasms occur in several different epilepsy syndromes and many different aetiologies have been described. Overall, the long-term outcome for cognitive development and for epilepsy control is poor. However, there is a small group of children whose spasms come under control rapidly and have a good long-term outcome (Vigevano et al., 1993; Dulac and Plouin, 1994). The first-line agents for treatment of infantile spasms are vigabatrin or steroids. Benzodiazepines are not usually considered until a trial of one or both of these agents has failed. In general, if spasms have not come under control after vigabatrin and/or prednisolone (or adrenocorticotropic hormone), it is unlikely that long-term control will be achieved. In this situation, benzodiazepines will often produce a temporary response but long-term control is unlikely. In children with idiopathic spasms, rapid seizure control is likely to have occurred with first- or second-line agents and so benzodiazepines will not usually have been used.

Largely for historical reasons, nitrazepam has been the most widely used benzodiazepine for infantile spasms (see above), and there is some suggestion that it may be more effective than clonazepam.

Lennox–Gastaut syndrome and other epileptic encephalopathies

The Lennox–Gastaut syndrome is one of the most drug-resistant and severe forms of childhood epilepsy. The precise nosological limits of this syndrome are the subject of continued debate; however, a core syndrome can readily be defined. Lennox–Gastaut syndrome is a severe childhood epilepsy characterized by frequent seizures of several different types. Most commonly these are atypical absences, tonic seizures and various forms of epileptic drop attacks. A characteristic EEG is associated with this syndrome. The interictal record often shows continuous or near-continuous generalized, irregular, slow spike and wave activity (1–2.5 cycles per second). The sleep EEG often shows bursts of bilateral rapid spike activity (10–20 cycles per second). These may be accompanied by tonic seizures and are highly suggestive of Lennox–Gastaut syndrome. The seizures are often very drug-resistant, and severe cognitive impairment, and often regression, occurs. This syndrome is therefore often referred to as a form of epileptic encephalopathy. Other severe childhood epilepsies can cause a similar clinical picture and there is overlap with some forms of myoclonic epilepsy, severe polymorphous epilepsy and so-called myoclonic astatic epilepsy. The newer antiepileptic agents have generally been tried early in this group of patients because of the severity of their epilepsy. There have therefore been reports of the use of nitrazepam, clonazepam and clobazam in the treatment of Lennox–Gastaut syndrome. As discussed above, the benzodiazepines often produce a dramatic response in these children, with efficacy against atypical absences, drop attacks and other seizure types. Clinical response is often striking with not only cessation of seizures but a marked cognitive improvement also. Unfortunately, tolerance frequently develops and behavioural side effects are common. Continued long-term response is rare. These drugs can, however, provide up to 6 months or longer of good seizure control. When tolerance develops, the drug should be withdrawn (see Table 1). After a drug holiday, reintroduction of the benzodiazepine may once more be effective.

Other epilepsy syndromes

The use of benzodiazepines should be considered in any drug-resistant epilepsy syndrome. Clobazam and clonazepam may both be effective in drug-resistant absence epilepsy but they would not normally be considered until after valproate, lamotrigine and ethosuximide have failed. Drug-resistant partial seizures may also respond. As with the epilepsy syndromes discussed above long-term response is rare.

MONOTHERAPY VERSUS ADD-ON THERAPY

Most often, benzodiazepines are used as add-on treatment. Because of their high rate of side effects there is a particular risk of the problems associated with polytherapy. There is no doubt, however, that monotherapy is possible with all of the currently used benzodiazepines. In the severe epilepsy syndromes of childhood, however, it is usually difficult to wean the child off all treatment prior to starting the benzodiazepine. The optimal situation is for the benzodiazepine to be added to one anchor drug.

Because of the problems with tolerance and the adverse effects of benzo-diazepines, alternative dosing strategies have been employed in an attempt to overcome this. There have been no systematic studies comparing these dose regimes to more conventional approaches. Alternate day benzodiazepines have been employed but this regime does not always prevent the development of tolerance.

Because of these problems benzodiazepines are increasingly used as intermittent treatments. This is considered in more detail elsewhere in this volume. In children, however, intermittent benzodiazepines may be very effective in the following situations:

1. Cluster epilepsy – many children will have predictable clusters of seizures, which will sometimes build up and eventually culminate in true status epilepticus. Provided they are able to take an oral medication, administration of clobazam 0.5–1 mg/kg early in the cluster may successfully abort it. If the child is unable to swallow tablets then sublingual or intranasal benzodiazepines may be effective (see below).
2. Some children have situation-related epilepsy and in these contexts a single oral dose of benzodiazepine prior to encountering the provoking situation may be effective.
3. Catamenial epilepsy in adolescence may be managed effectively by intermittent benzodiazepines.

STATUS EPILEPTICUS

Benzodiazepines are generally considered as a first-line treatment for all types of status epilepticus in children as well as adults (Delgado-Escueta *et al.*, 1990; Epilepsy Foundation of America Working Group on Status Epilepticus, 1993; Livingston, 1996). Diazepam will control status epilepticus in 80% of patients within 5 minutes of administration (Treiman, 1990). Because of its short duration of action diazepam is not effective as a single agent and needs to be given with a longer-acting AED such as phenytoin. Lorazepam has a longer duration of action than diazepam and comparative studies have shown it to be as effective as other benzodiazepines and phenytoin (Leppik *et al.*, 1983; Crawford *et al.*, 1987; Treiman, 1990). For this reason many protocols now recommend lorazepam as first-line treatment.

Clonazepam is as effective as diazepam in the control of status epilepticus but it appears to have no particular advantage over diazepam. In the 1980s, there was a vogue for treating status epilepticus with continuous infusions of benzodiazepines. There appears to be no particular advantage to this regimen over bolus treatment. Adverse effects in the form of respiratory depression and sedation, however, are common.

Midazolam is an extremely potent short-acting benzodiazepine that has been used to treat status epilepticus (Kumar and Bleck 1992; Parent and Lowenstein, 1994). Midazolam has been most often used in the intensive care context when the patient is already intubated and ventilated. It is, however, effectively absorbed by the intramuscular route and this may be an advantage in a plump infant in whom venous access has not been established.

NON-CONVULSIVE STATUS EPILEPTICUS

Non-convulsive status epilepticus is increasingly recognized in childhood as a cause of acute, subacute or chronic behavioural change (Stores, 1986). The most common form in childhood is atypical absence status epilepticus. Complex partial status epilepticus is much less common and typical absence status epilepticus is rare in childhood. First-line treatment for all of these forms of status epilepticus is intravenous benzodiazepines. Complex partial status epilepticus and typical absence status epilepticus respond well to benzodiazepines (Mayeux and Lueders, 1978; Porter and Penry, 1983; Treiman and Delgado-Escueta, 1983). Atypical absence status epilepticus, however, is often quite resistant to treatment and has a much lower response rate to benzodiazepines than any other form of status epilepticus (Tassinari et al., 1983; Livingston and Brown, 1987). In Lennox–Gastaut syndrome, intravenous benzodiazepines can precipitate tonic status epilepticus (Prior et al., 1972; Tassinari et al., 1972). As atypical absence status epilepticus is a common component of Lennox–Gastaut syndrome this is a significant risk.

OTHER USES OF BENZODIAZEPINES IN CHILDHOOD EPILEPSY

Rectal diazepam

Diazepam administered rectally is rapidly absorbed, reaching peak levels within 4–11 minutes (Knudsen, 1977; Moolenar et al., 1980). It has become widely used in paediatric practice since the early 1980s in the termination of prolonged seizures and prevention of status epilepticus. Rectal diazepam is used by both medical and non-medical personnel as first aid treatment in a child prior to admission to hospital; this is undoubtedly one of the factors in the reduced incidence of very prolonged status epilepticus and its consequences such as hemiconvulsion, hemiplegia epilepsy syndrome (Gross-Tsur and Shinnar, 1993). In many countries, diazepam is available as a specific rectal preparation enabling rapid and easy administration. The major role of rectal diazepam is in pre-hospital treatment of prolonged seizures. Because it may have erratic absorption and sometimes delayed effects it is not recommended for the treatment of status epilepticus in hospital unless venous access is not established.

Rectal diazepam may also be effective in the same situations as intermittent oral benzodiazepines, such as cluster epilepsy or certain situation-related seizure types. It is clearly more acceptable to the patient and family to treat these types of seizures with oral benzodiazepines rather than rectal preparations. In recent years other routes of administration have been employed and shown to be effective, such as sublingual and intranasal use of midazolam (O'Regan *et al.*, 1996; Scott *et al.*, 1998) and sublingual lorazepam (Yager and Seshia, 1988). These may be as effective as rectal diazepam.

SUMMARY

The benzodiazepines are potent antiepileptic agents with activity against most seizure types. They have a relatively high rate of behavioural and cognitive side effects and a strong tendency to cause withdrawal seizures on over-rapid dose reduction or cessation. Tolerance to their effects occurs in a significant proportion of patients. For these reasons benzodiazepines are most useful as intermittent or acute treatment for status epilepticus or clustering of epileptic seizures.

Chronic oral benzodiazepine therapy is usually considered for drug-resistant childhood epilepsy such as infantile spasms, myoclonic astatic epilepsy and Lennox–Gastaut syndrome. In these syndromes, benzodiazepines are often effective as third- or fourth-line agents as add-on therapy. Although response may be transient, sustained responses do occur. Benzodiazepines may also be effective as add-on therapy in other poorly controlled epilepsy syndromes and against partial or absence seizures.

Clobazam is currently the preferred benzodiazepine for oral treatment of epilepsy, although few comparative studies of different benzodiazepines have been performed.

A recent multicentre study in newly diagnosed or recent onset epilepsy suggests that clobazam may be well tolerated and effective as monotherapy. It was, however, no more effective than carbamazepine or phenytoin.

Unless the problem of tolerance, adverse effects and withdrawal seizures can be circumvented, benzodiazepines are unlikely to become first- or second-line AEDs in childhood epilepsy. However, in spite of the new AEDs of the last decade, benzodiazepines maintain an important overall place in the drug treatment of childhood epilepsy.

REFERENCES

Allen, J.W., Oxley, J., Robertson, M.M., Trimble, M., Richens, A. and Jawad, S. (1983). Clobazam as adjunctive treatment in refractory epilepsy. *BMJ* **286**, 1246–1247.

Andre, M., Boutroy, M.J., Biachetti, G., Vert, P. and Morselli, P.L. (1991). Clonazepam in neonatal seizures: dose regimens and therapeutic efficacy. *Eur J Clin Pharmacol* **40**, 193–195.

Bourgeois, B.F.D. (1996). Antiepileptic drugs. In: Wallace, S. (ed.) *Epilepsy in Children*. Chapman and Hall, London, pp. 544–546.

Browne, T.R. (1976). Clonazepam: a review of a new anticonvulsant drug. *Arch Neurol* **33**, 326–332.

Browne, T.R. (1983). Benzodiazepines. In: Browne, T.R. and Feldman, R.G. (Eds), *Epilepsy: Diagnosis and Management*. Raven Press, New York, pp. 235–245.

Browne, T.R. and Penry, J.K. (1973). Benzodiazepines in the treatment of epilepsy. *Epilepsia* **14**, 277–310.

Burdette, D.E. and Browne, T.R. (1990). Benzodiazepines. In: Dam, M. and Gram, L. (Eds), *Comprehensive Epileptology*. Raven Press, New York, pp. 547–561.

Canadian Clobazam Co-operative Group (1990). Clobazam in the treatment of refractory epilepsy: the Canadian experience. *Epilepsia* **32**, 407–415.

Canadian Study Group for Childhood Epilepsy (1998). Clobazam has equivalent efficacy to carbamazepine and phenytoin as monotherapy for childhood epilepsy. *Epilepsia* **39**, 952–959.

Carson, M. (1968). Treatment of minor motor seizures with nitrazepam. *Dev Med Child Neurol* **10**, 772–775.

Crawford, T.O., Mitchell, W.G. and Snodgrass, S.R. (1987). Lorazepam in childhood status epilepticus and serial seizures: effectiveness and tachyphylaxis. *Neurology* **37**, 190–195.

Delgado-Escueta, A.V., Swartz, B. and Abad-Herrera, P. (1990). Status epilepticus. In: Dam, M. and Gram, L. (Eds), *Comprehensive Epileptology*. Raven Press, New York, pp. 251–270.

Dreifuss, F.E., Penry, J.K., Rose, S.W., Kupferberg, H.J., Dyken, P. and Sato, S. (1975) Serum clonazepam concentrations in children with absence seizures. *Neurology* **23**, 255–258.

Dreifuss, F., Farwell, J., Holmes, G. *et al.* (1986). Infantile spasms: comparative trial of nitrazepam and corticotrophin. *Arch Neurol* **43**, 1107–1110.

Dulac, O. and Plouin, P. (1994). Cryptogenic/idiopathic West syndrome. In: Dulac, O., Chugani, H.T. and Della Bernardina, B. (Eds), *Infantile spasms and West Syndrome*. WB Saunders, London, pp. 232–243.

Epilepsy Foundation of America Working Group on Status Epilepticus (1993). Treatment of convulsive status epilepticus. *JAMA* **270**, 854–859.

Farrell, K. (1986). Benzodiazepines in the treatment of children with epilepsy. *Epilepsia* **27** (suppl 1), S45–S51.

Gastaut, H. (1978). Proprietes antiepileptique exceptionelles et meconnues d'un anxiolytique du commerce, le Clobazam. *Concours Med* **100**, 3697–3701.

Gross-Tsur, V. and Shinnar, S. (1993). Convulsive status epilepticus in children. *Epilepsia* **34** (suppl 1), S12–S20.

Haigh, J.R.M. and Feely, M. (1988). Tolerance to the anticonvulsant effect of benzo-diazepines. *Trends Pharmacol Sci* **9**, 298–303.

Ishikawa, A., Sakuma, N., Nagashima, T., Kohsaka, S. and Kajii, N. (1985). Clonazepam monotherapy for epilepsy in childhood. *Brain Dev* **7**, 610–613.

Keene, D.L., Whiting, S. and Humphreys, P. (1990). Clobazam as an add-on drug in the treatment of refractory epilepsy in childhood. *J Neurol Sci* **17**, 317–319.

Knudsen, F.U. (1977). Plasma–diazepam in infants after rectal administration in solution and by suppository. *Acta Paediatr Scand* **66**, 563–567.

Ko, D.Y., Rho, J.M., DeGiorgio, C.M. and Sato, S. (1997). Benzodiazepines. In:

Engel, J. Jr and Pedley, T.A. (Eds), *Epilepsy: A Comprehensive Textbook*. Lippincott-Raven, Philadelphia, pp. 1475–1490.

Koeppen, D. (1985). A review of clobazam studies in epilepsy. In: Hindmarch, I., Stonier, P.D. and Trimble, M.R. (Eds), *Clobazam: Human Psychopharmacology and Clinical Applications*. London: Royal Society of Medicine International Congress and Symposium Series, **74**, 207–215.

Kumar, A. and Bleck, T.P. (1992). Intravenous midazolam for the treatment of refractory status epilepticus. *Crit Care Med* **20**, 483–488.

Leppik, I.E., Derivan, A.T., Homan, R.W., Walker, J., Ramsey, E. and Patrick, B. (1983). Double-blind study of lorazepam and diazepam in status epilepticus. *JAMA* **249**, 1452–1454.

Liske, E. and Forster, F.M. (1963). Clinical study of a new benzodiazepine as an anticonvulsant agent. *J New Drugs* **3**, 241–244.

Livingston, J. (1996). Status epilepticus. In: Wallace, S. (Ed), *Epilepsy in Children*. Chapman and Hall, London, pp. 429–448.

Livingston, J.H. and Brown, J.K. (1987). Non-convulsive status epilepticus resistant to benzodiazepines. *Arch Dis Child* **62**, 41–44.

Lund, M and Trolle, E. (1973). Clonazepam in the treatment of epilepsy. *Acta Neurol Scand* **49** (Suppl 53), 82–90.

Mayeux, R. and Lueders, H. (1978) Complex partial status epilepticus, case report and proposal for diagnostic criteria. *Neurology* **28**, 657–661.

Meldrum, B.S. and Croucher, M.J. (1982). Anticonvulsant action of clobazam and desmethyl clobazam in reflex epilepsy in rodents and baboons. *Drug Dev Res* **1** (Suppl), 33–38.

Millichap, J.G. and Ortiz, W.R. (1966). Nitrazepam in myoclonic epilepsies. *Am J Dis Child* **112**, 242–248.

Moolenar, F., Bakker, S., Visser, J. and Huizinga, T. (1980). Biopharmaceutics of rectal administration of drugs in man. IX. Comparative biopharmaceutics of diazepam after single rectal, oral, intramuscular and intravenous administration in man. *Int J Pharmaceutics* **5**, 127–137.

O'Donohoe, N.V. and Paes, B.A. (1977). A trial of clonazepam in the treatment of severe epilepsy in infancy and childhood. In: Penry, J.K. (Ed), *Epilepsy: the VIIIth International Symposium*. Raven Press, New York, pp. 159–162.

O'Regan, M.E., Brown, J.K. and Clarke, M. (1996). Nasal rather than rectal benzodiazepines in the management of acute childhood seizures? *Dev Med Child Neurol* **38**, 1037–1045.

Parent, J.M. and Lowenstein, D.H. (1994). Treatment of refractory generalised status epilepticus with a continuous infusion of midazolam. *Neurology* **44**, 1837–1840.

Porter, R.J. and Penry, J.K. (1983). Petit mal status. *Adv Neurol* **34**, 61–68.

Prior, P.F., McLaine, G.N., Scott, D.F. and Laurance, B.M. (1972). Tonic status epilepticus precipitated by intravenous diazepam in a child with petit mal status. *Epilepsia* **13**, 467–472.

Reider, J and Wendt, G. (1973). Pharmacokinetics and metabolism of the hypnotic nitrazepam. In: Garattini, S., Mussini, E. and Randall, L.O. (Eds), *The Benzodiazepines*. Raven Press, New York, pp. 99–127.

Remy, C. (1994). Clobazam in the treatment of epilepsy: a review of the literature. *Epilepsia* **35** (suppl 5), S88–S91.

Robertson, M.M. (1986). Current status of the 1,4 and 1,5-benzodiazepines in the treatment of epilepsy: the place of clobazam. *Epilepsia* **27** (suppl 1), 527–541.

Schmidt, D. (1983). How to use benzodiazepines. In: Morselli, P.L., Pippenger, C.E.

and Penry, J.K. (Eds), *Antiepileptic Drug Therapy in Paediatrics*. Raven Press, New York, pp. 271–278.

Schmidt, D. (1985). Benzodiazepine – an update. In: Pedley, T.A. and Meldrum, B.S. (Eds), *Recent Advances in Epilepsy, Vol. 2*. Churchill Livingstone, Edinburgh, pp. 125–135.

Schmidt, D. (1994). Clobazam for treatment of intractable epilepsy: a critical assessment. *Epilepsia* **35** (suppl 5), S92–S95.

Schmidt, D., Rohde, M., Wolf, P. and Roeder-Wanner, U. (1986a). Clobazam for refractory epilepsy: a controlled trial. *Arch Neurol* **43**, 824–826.

Schmidt, D., Rohde, M., Wolf, P. and Roeder-Wanner, U. (1986b). Tolerance to the antiepileptic effect of clobazam. In: Koella, W. P., Frey, H.H., Froscher, W. and Meinardi, H. (Eds), *Tolerance to Beneficial and Adverse Effects of Antiepileptic Drugs*. Raven Press, New York, pp. 109–115.

Schoch, P., Moreau, J.L., Martin, J.R. and Haefely, W.E. (1993). Aspects of benzodiazepine structure and function with relevance to drug tolerance and dependence. *Biochem Soc Symp* **59**, 121–134.

Scott, R.C., Besag, F.M., Boyd, S.G., Berry, D. and Neville, B.G. (1998). Buccal absorption of midazolam: pharmacokinetics and EEG pharmacodynamics. *Epilepsia* **39**, 290–294.

Sheth, R.D., Ronen, G.M., Goulden, K.J., Penney, S. and Bodensteiner, J.B. (1995). Clobazam for intractable pediatric epilepsy. *J Child Neurol* **10**, 205–208.

Singh, A., Guberman, A.H. and Boisvert, D. (1995). Clobazam in long-term epilepsy treatment: sustained responders versus those developing tolerance. *Epilepsia* **36**, 798–803

Stores, G. (1986). Non-convulsive status epilepticus. In: Pedley, T.A. and Meldrum, B.S. (Eds), *Recent Advances in Epilepsy 3*. Churchill Livingstone, Edinburgh, pp. 295–310.

Tassinari, C.A., Dravet, C., Roger, J., Cano, J.P. and Gastaut, H. (1972). Tonic status epilepticus precipitated by intravenous benzodiazepine in five patients with Lennox–Gastaut syndrome. *Epilepsia* **13**, 421–435.

Tassinari, C.A., Daniele, O., Michelucci, R., Bureau, M., Dravet, C. and Roger, J. (1983). Benzodiazepines: efficacy in status epilepticus. *Adv Neurol* **34**, 465–475.

Theis, J.G.W., Koren, G., Daneman, R., Sherwin, A.L. Menzano, E., Cortez, M. and Hwang, P. (1997) Interactions of clobazam with conventional antiepileptics in children. *J Child Neurol* **12**, 208–213.

Treiman, D.M. (1990). The role of benzodiazepines in the management of status epilepticus. *Neurology* **40**, (suppl 2), 32–42.

Treiman, D.M. and Delgado-Escueta, A.V. (1983). Complex partial status epilepticus. *Adv Neurol* **34**, 69–82.

Vasella, F., Pavlincova, E., Schneider, H.J., Rudin, H.J. and Karbowski, K. (1973). Treatment of infantile spasms and Lennox–Gastaut syndrome with clonazepam. *Epilepsia* **14**, 165–175.

Vigevano, F., Fusco, L., Cusmai, R., Claps, D., Ricci, S. and Milani, L. (1993). The idiopathic form of West syndrome. *Epilepsia* **34**, 743–746.

Yager, J.Y. and Seshia, S.S. (1988). Sublingual lorazepam in childhood serial seizures. *Am J Dis Child* **142**, 931–932.

Benzodiazepines
Edited by Michael R. Trimble and Ian Hindmarch
© 2000 Wrightson Biomedical Publishing Ltd

9

Tolerance to the Antiepileptic Action of Clobazam

ALAN GUBERMAN

Division of Neurology, University of Ottawa, The Ottawa Hospital, Ottawa, Ontario, Canada

INTRODUCTION

Benzodiazepines, in addition to their anxiolytic, sedative–hypnotic and muscle relaxant effects, are powerful antiepileptic drugs effective against a variety of chemically and electrically induced seizures in animal models (Shrader and Greenblatt, 1993; Shorvon, 1995). Their long-term clinical use, however, has been largely limited by their sedative properties and the development of tolerance, which leads to loss of effectiveness over time in many cases. In epilepsy practice, they are most often employed acutely to treat status epilepticus or intermittently to treat serial seizures or seizures occurring in specific situations such as with alcohol withdrawal or febrile convulsions in children.

Clobazam is a benzodiazepine with the two nitrogens located at the 1,5 position of the diazepine ring in comparison to the 1,4 position in other clinically used benzodiazepines. It also has an active N-desmethyl metabolite which is partially responsible for its antiepileptic properties (Robertson, 1986; 1995). Clobazam was first released as an anxiolytic in Europe in the 1970s but began to be used as an antiepileptic drug about 20 years ago. It is less sedating and a stronger anticonvulsant than the 1,4-benzodiazepines (Hindmarch, 1995). Numerous open and controlled double-blind trials in adults and children have proven it to be a well-tolerated and effective agent for a variety of seizure types, both as an adjuvant agent and in monotherapy (Schmidt, 1994; Robertson, 1995; Shorvon, 1995).

Although a relatively high incidence of tolerance has relegated clobazam to a second- or third-line agent for epilepsy and has contributed to the fact that it has not been released in the USA, the data concerning tolerance have been quite inconsistent. Several recent studies have attempted to better characterize the phenomenon. The purpose of this chapter is to present data on tolerance with clobazam, to discuss some of the reasons for the conflicting data, to mention the unsuccessful strategies that have been tried to forestall or overcome tolerance and to touch on some of the experimental data relating to possible mechanisms of tolerance.

DEFINITION AND CHARACTERISTICS OF TOLERANCE

Tolerance has been defined as: 'a reduction over time in one or more pharmacologic effects as a consequence of continued drug use attributable to a decrease in receptor sensitivity' (Shrader and Greenblatt, 1993). In other words, tolerance is a loss of efficacy of a drug over time that is not due to a reduction in blood or central nervous system levels. It is a pharmacodynamic rather than a pharmacokinetic phenomenon. Selective tolerance to only some of the pharmacologic effects of a drug may occur or tolerance to various drug effects may occur at different rates (Rosenberg et al., 1989). For example, tolerance to the sedative effect of benzodiazepines may occur at a time when the anticonvulsant effects are preserved. This may be due to differential effects on gamma-aminobutyric acid (GABA) receptors from different brain regions reflecting different subunit composition. Tolerance may be complete (i.e. total loss of the drug effect) or only partial. In many clinical studies with clobazam in epilepsy there has been a failure to distinguish between complete and partial tolerance. It is also possible for tolerance in experimental models to occur with respect to some seizure types when efficacy for other seizure types is preserved or only to certain components of a particular seizure type. In experimental models, tolerance to the anticonvulsant effects of benzodiazepines developed more readily in some models than in others (Rosenberg et al., 1989; Wildin and Pleuvry, 1992; Rundfeldt et al., 1995; Loscher et al., 1996).

Benzodiazepines have been classified into three main categories: full allosteric modulators (FAM) at the GABA-A receptor complex (e.g. triazolam, flurazepam, lorazepam); partial allosteric modulators (PAM) such as imidazenil and bretazenil; and antagonists such as flumazenil. Inverse agonists, both partial and full, have also been discovered but have not been developed clinically. Tolerance develops with FAMs, much less readily with PAMs (Ghiani et al., 1994) and not at all with antagonists. It is unclear whether clobazam is an FAM or PAM (Malizia and Nutt, 1995), but tolerance has been shown to develop more rapidly to clobazam in experimental models of epilepsy than to other benzodiazepines such as clonazepam or diazepam and even N-D-clobazam (Rosenberg et al., 1989; De Sarro et al., 1996). In fact, flumazenil may reverse experimental tolerance to FAMs

(Savic *et al.*, 1991). There is cross reactivity for tolerance to benzodiazepines of the same class (Haigh and Feely, 1988). These features support the concept that tolerance is due to specific changes occurring at the GABA receptor complex which reduce its sensitivity to the drug (Itier *et al.*, 1996).

POSSIBLE MECHANISMS OF TOLERANCE OF BENZODIAZEPINES

The precise mechanism for the development of decreased sensitivity of the GABA-A receptor complex to benzodiazepines over time is unknown. It has been suggested that tolerance represents simple GABA-A receptor down-regulation although there is evidence against this (Barnes, 1996). Reduced coupling between GABA-A receptor/chloride channel gating and benzodi-azepine receptor binding is another proposed mechanism for tolerance. Recent experimental evidence in various animal models of acute seizures points to changes in the regional distribution of GABA-A receptor subunit composition over time as the likely mechanism for tolerance (Tietz *et al.*, 1993; Impagnatiello *et al.*, 1996; Ramsey-Williams and Carter, 1996; Pesold *et al.*, 1997; Chen *et al.*, 1999).

The GABA-A receptor complex is a pentomer of peptide subunits (at least 16 varieties), derived from α, β, γ, δ classes, which incorporates the chloride channel. There are benzodiazepine, neurosteroid, barbiturate and picrotoxin modulatory sites on the receptor complex. Benzodiazepine receptors are located on the α (especially $\alpha1$) subunit and the GABA-A recognition, barbi-turate, picrotoxin and neurosteroid sites on the β subunit. Benzodiazepine binding also appears to require a $\gamma2$ subunit.

In rats treated with flurazepam for 4 weeks, there is a reduction in $\beta2$ and $\beta3$ GABA-A subunit mRNAs in cerebellum and hippocampus and reduc-tion of $\beta2$ in cortex. Reduction in $\beta3$ subunit mRNA is seen in cortex 4 hours after single-dose flurazepam treatment (Zhao *et al.*, 1994).

In rats made tolerant to diazepam effects on bicuculline-induced seizures, mRNA encoding for the $\alpha1$ subunit of the GABA-A receptor was reduced in the frontoparietal cortex and hippocampus (Impagnatiello *et al.*, 1996). Rats made tolerant to the anticonvulsant effect of diazepam on bicuculline-induced seizures had GABA-A receptor subunits measured by immuno-histochemistry in the frontoparietal motor and somatosensory cortex. There was a reduction in the expression of $\alpha1$ and increase in $\alpha5$, $\gamma2$ and $\beta2/3$ subunits. No significant changes were seen with the partial allosteric modula-tor imidazenil, which did not produce tolerance (Pesold *et al.*, 1997).

Immunohistochemical staining of GABA-A receptor subunits in rats given flurazepam chronically shows a decrease in $\alpha1$ and $\beta3$ subunit density in hippocampus and certain cortical regions. Gamma-2 subunit density was reduced only in the dentate gyrus (Chen *et al.*, 1999). These and other studies suggest that tolerance may be explained by regional changes in GABA-A receptor subpopulations over time, which render them less sensitive to benzodiazepines.

TOLERANCE TO CLOBAZAM IN CLINICAL STUDIES

Clobazam, but not *N*-desmethylclobazam, demonstrated tolerance more readily than clonazepam in the rat pentylenetetrazol seizure model (Haigh and Feely, 1988) and clobazam also produced tolerance more quickly than clonazepam or diazepam in amygdala-kindled rats (Rosenberg *et al.*, 1989; De Sarro *et al.*, 1996). Early clinical European studies summarized by Remy (1994), Schmidt (1994), Robertson (1986; 1995) and Shorvon (1995) showed widely varying estimates of tolerance ranging from 23% to 89% (mean 45 ± 27%) (Remy, 1994) in studies of at least 1 year in duration.

How can the wide variation among studies in the incidence of tolerance with clobazam be explained? The problem with interpreting these incidence figures is that they are derived from studies with widely different methodologies and durations. Furthermore, serum levels are not often obtained to rule out a decline in blood levels as an explanation for loss of efficacy. More importantly, the definition of tolerance is often either not specified or variable from study to study. There is no universally accepted definition of tolerance to antiepileptic drugs in clinical practice. Most clinicians would agree that tolerance involves a significant escape from response of seizures to the antiepileptic drug over time, but problems arise in attempting to define the duration of seizure-free interval necessary, following initiation of therapy, which would indicate a response to the drug and what degree of relapse is necessary to constitute tolerance.

The problem can be illustrated by a theoretical patient who is having an average of one seizure a week for the 6 months prior to addition of clobazam. After clobazam is added, the patient remains seizure-free for 4 weeks and then has one seizure every 2 weeks for the next 4 months. Does this patient's course illustrate tolerance or just natural variation in seizure frequency?

Central to a clinical definition of tolerance are:

1. Determination of the baseline seizure frequency or mean interseizure interval of the patient prior to treatment. The necessary baseline period will vary according to the seizure frequency.
2. Determination of the degree of response to the drug because tolerance will only apply to patients who actually respond to the drug. A prolongation of the mean baseline seizure interval by at least three- to five-fold can be considered as an indication of response. This response should be

maintained over a specified period of time.
3. Definition of what degree of relapse over what period of time constitutes an escape from response (i.e. tolerance).
4. Control for stability of serum levels for both the test drug and concurrent antiepileptic drugs.

Despite the pitfalls of determining tolerance, there are patients who show a dramatic response to clobazam and become seizure-free, perhaps for the first time, over a period of several pretreatment mean seizure intervals, and then relapse to their former seizure frequency. It is in such patients that clinicians feel most confident in applying the term tolerance. It is also such patients who often become extremely disheartened when they relapse after having been given false hope by a new, initially successful, treatment.

Several recent clinical studies with clobazam have tried to look at the tolerance issue. These studies have attempted to determine both the incidence of and predictors for tolerance. Bardy and colleagues (1991) in Finland studied 90 children (median age 6.4 years) who had clobazam added to their antiepilpetic drug regimen (7/90 monotherapy) due to intractable epilepsy. Patients were followed for at least 1 year or to the point of clobazam withdrawal. Six patients (7%) had sustained freedom from all seizures. Four of these patients developed tolerance after 4–40 weeks of complete seizure control. Of 33 additional patients experiencing ≥50% seizure reduction, 24 developed tolerance. Tolerance was defined as an initial freedom from, or decrease (≥50% reduction) in seizures followed by an 'unchanged' seizure frequency. No time intervals for these determinations were specified. Tolerance occurred in 65% of patients overall with a range of 4–40 weeks (median 8 weeks), and did not appear to be related to low serum levels. An increase in dose (two patients) or temporary drug holiday (four patients) did not restore response to clobazam.

Munn and Farrell (1993) conducted a prospective open add-on trial of clobazam in 114 paediatric (<18 years) patients with intractable epilepsy. Follow-up was for a minimum of 5 months and a mean of 18 months. Most of the patients had multiple, resistant seizure types and 25 had Lennox–Gastaut syndrome. Eighteen (16%) patients followed for at least 5 months became seizure-free, an additional 35 (31%) had ≥90% improvement and 17 (15%) had a ≥50% improvement. Tolerance (loosely defined) developed in 30 out of 79 (38%) of the responders after 2–24 months (mean 7 months, median 3 months). Out of 30 patients, tolerance was complete in nine, was partial in nine and in 12 'tolerance' responded to an increase in dose.

A Canadian study pooled the retrospective data from 32 neurologists who had used clobazam as an add-on agent for ≥10 patients through a compassionate release programme between 1982 and 1989 (Canadian Clobazam Cooperative Group, 1990). Data were available for 424 adults (≥16 years),

440 children and 13 with age unspecified out of a total of 1319 patients treated. All seizure types were represented and complex partial seizures were seen in 43.9% of the patients. Remarkably, retention rates on clobazam were 70% at 1 year and 40–50% at 4 years. These rates must be viewed with a realization that none of the other newer antiepileptic drugs had been marketed in Canada at the time. Tolerance (not defined) was given as a reason for discontinuation by the treating physician in only 81 out of 877 (9.2%), suggesting that it was not a major problem. Of the 81 patients judged to have shown tolerance, 43 out of 81 occurred within the first year of treatment.

Buchanan (1995) conducted a long-term (up to 11 years) open study of clobazam, added to or substituted for standard antiepileptic drugs in 90 patients: both children and adults. Partial epilepsy was present in 63 patients, primary generalized in seven patients and secondarily generalized with mental retardation in 20 patients. Clobazam was the sole antiepileptic drug in 57.8% of cases. Fourteen of 90 patients became seizure-free and an additional four had ≥90% seizure reduction. However, clobazam was discontinued in 63 out of 90 (70%) of the patients. Tolerance (not defined) was seen in 17 out of 90 (18.8%) and in 9 out of 11 seizure-free patients. The mean time to develop tolerance was 8.5 ± 3 months (range 2–36 months).

The development of tolerance was examined retrospectively in a series of 173 consecutively treated adult patients who had clobazam added to their baseline antiepileptic drugs (Singh et al., 1995). These patients had largely longstanding partial epilepsy and four or more seizures per month. Of 173 patients treated, 50 were identified as very good responders with ≥75% seizure reduction. It is only in these patients that tolerance was examined according to the following definition:

1. Treatment for at least 1 month.
2. No evidence for non-compliance or fall in serum levels of clobazam (where levels were measured).
3. Relapse to at least 50% of the pre-clobazam seizure frequency.

Some 50% of the excellent responders developed tolerance after a mean of 8.9 months (mean follow-up of 17 ± 15.7 months in this group). Of the 25 patients developing tolerance, only 44% discontinued the drug, suggesting only partial tolerance in about half the group. Of the 25 patients whose response was maintained, the mean follow-up was 37.3 ± 12.8 months. Several parameters were compared in the tolerance versus the sustained-response group. The only significant differences were higher incidence of known aetiology (also seen by Heller et al., 1988), higher serum clobazam (but not N-D-clobazam) levels, and a longer duration of epilepsy in the tolerance group. Despite the 50% incidence of tolerance according to the above definition, almost 15% of the total patients treated continued to show a sustained long-term very good response to clobazam.

Sultan and colleagues (personal communication, 1996) performed a retro-spective review of patients treated with clobazam (add-on) for epilepsy at the Montreal Neurological Hospital, which was very similar to that by Singh and colleagues (1995). However, responders in this study were defined as having ≥50% seizure reduction. As with Singh and colleagues, tolerance was clearly defined and plasma levels were measured to ensure stability. Tolerance was seen in 23 out of 75 (30.6%) patients after a mean of 10.8 months (range 3.5–21 months). Similarly to Singh and colleagues, 17 out of 23 patients continued to benefit and remain on clobazam. There were no discernible differences between sustained responders and the group developing tolerance.

A recent well-designed, double-blind multicentre, paediatric study compared clobazam ($n = 119$) to either carbamazepine ($n = 37$) or pheny-toin ($n = 79$) in monotherapy (Canadian Study Group for Childhood Epilepsy, 1998). There were 209 patients with partial and 26 with primary generalized epilepsy. All were either naive to treatment or had failed one drug, indicating that they were relatively mild cases. Doses were adjusted blindly according to seizure response and reports of blood level ranges, mimicking clinical practice as closely as possible. Efficacy, judged by 12-month retention rates, was equal for the three drugs: 55% on clobazam, 65% on carbamazepine and 39% on phenytoin. Side effects, including somnolence and behavioural change, did not differ among the three drugs.

Tolerance was carefully defined as breakthrough seizures sufficient to lead to discontinuation after a seizure-free period (defined as at least three times the pretreatment inter-seizure interval during baseline) in patients treated for at least 3 months. Of the patients eligible for tolerance calculation, 4 out of 53 (7.5%) developed it on clobazam, 2 out of 48 (4.2%) on carbamazepine and 1 out of 15 (6.7%) on phenytoin. The relatively low figure for tolerance on clobazam in this study is probably related to at least four factors: the fairly mild nature of the epilepsy in these patients in comparison with the intractable cases treated in most other studies; the requirement for 3 months of treatment, which eliminates patients who develop early tolerance; the use of discontinuation or relapse as a measurement of tolerance rather than a comparison of seizure frequencies; and termination of the study after 12 months, which would miss late cases of tolerance.

These studies, some of them more carefully conducted than the earlier studies with clobazam, suggest that significant loss of response to clobazam over time probably occurs in about one-quarter to one-half of patients. There are no reliable predictors of which patients are likely to develop tolerance. Tolerance, if it occurs, usually does so in the first year of treatment but can occur later. It must be recognized that many of the responders to clobazam will have a sustained response over several years.

Once tolerance to clobazam develops, there are no effective strategies to restore responsivity. Various manipulations have been tried including increasing the dose (Haigh *et al.*, 1988), or stopping and later restarting the drug. Strategies to forestall the development of tolerance including drug holidays have likewise been largely ineffective. Theoretically, administration of the weak benzodiazepine antagonist flumazenil may be able to reverse tolerance to the anticonvulsant effects of FAMs such as clobazam but there are limited clinical data attempting to apply this strategy (Savic *et al.*, 1991).

A recent Japanese study using nitrazepam in the pentylenetetrazol mouse model concluded that flunarizine (a calcium channel blocker), but not traditional anticonvulsants, administered with the benzodiazepine could prevent the development of tolerance (Suzuki *et al.*, 1998). Another experimental animal study suggested that concurrent neurosteroid administration might be able to prevent tolerance to the anxiolytic and sedative action of benzodiazepines (Reddy and Kulkarni, 1997). In specific groups of patients where intermittent treatment is necessary, tolerance is not an issue. Clobazam has been used successfully in catamenial epilepsy (Feely and Gibson, 1984, see also Chapter 10), in the treatment of febrile convulsions (Tondi *et al.*, 1987), in the management of partial status epilepticus with an oral loading dose of up to 70 mg (Corman *et al.*, 1998), and the present author and co-workers have used it for serial or 'cluster' seizures in patients with non-convulsive generalized status epilepticus and added to a patient's baseline antiepileptic drugs for occasional use to prevent seizures on special occasions.

CONCLUSIONS

These recent studies suggest that tolerance to clobazam, depending on how it is defined, develops in approximately one-quarter to one-half of patients but that a substantial proportion of patients, including some who develop partial tolerance, will continue to benefit from the drug. Up to 15% of uncontrolled partial-seizure patients who receive add-on clobazam will obtain a marked sustained reduction of seizures with complete control in approximately 10%. Tolerance may be even less of a problem in relatively mild cases and with monotherapy (Canadian Study Group for Childhood Epilepsy, 1998). Because of its effectiveness, broad spectrum, relatively low cost and excellent side effect profile, clobazam should be considered as the benzodiazepine of choice in chronic epilepsy treatment and as an early adjuvant agent for resistant partial epilepsy.

REFERENCES

Bardy, A.H., Seppälä, T., Salokorpi, T., Granström, M.-L. and Santavoori, P. (1991). Monitoring of concentrations of clobazam and norclobazam in serum and saliva of children with epilepsy. *Brain Dev* **13**, 174–179.

Barnes, E.M., Jr (1996). Use-dependent regulation of $GABA_A$ receptors. *Int Rev Neurobiol* **39**, 53–76.

Buchanan, N. (1995). Long-term follow-up to 11 years in adult and pediatric epilepsy. Presented at the 21st International Epilepsy Congress, Sydney, Australia.

Canadian Clobazam Cooperative Group (1990). Clobazam in the treatment of refractory epilepsy: the Canadian experience. A retrospective study. *Epilepsia* **32**, 407–415.

Canadian Study Group for Childhood Epilepsy (1998). Clobazam has equivalent efficacy to carbamazepine and phenytoin as monotherapy for childhood epilepsy. *Epilepsia* **39**, 952–959.

Chen, S., Huang, X., Zeng, X.J., Sieghart, W. and Tietz, E.I. (1999). Benzodiazepine – mediated regulation of alpha 1–2, beta 1–3 and gamma 2 GABAA receptor subunit proteins in the rat brain hippocampus and cortex. *Neuroscience* **93**, 33–44.

Corman, C., Guberman, A. and Benavente, O. (1998). Clobazam in partial status epilepticus. *Seizure* **7**, 243–248.

De Sarro, G., Di Paola, E.D., Aguglia, V. and de Sarro, A. (1996). Tolerance to anticonvulsant effects of benzodiazepines in genetically epilepsy-prone rats. *Pharmacol Biochem Behav* **55**, 39–48.

Feely, M. and Gibson, J. (1984). Intermittent clobazam for catamenial epilepsy: tolerance avoided. *J Neurol Neurosurg Psychiatry* **47**, 1279–1282.

Ghiani, C.A., Serra, M., Motzo, C. *et al.* (1994). Chronic administration of an anticonvulsant dose of imidazenil fails to induce tolerance of GABAA receptor functioning in mice. *Eur J Pharmacol* **254**, 299–302.

Haigh, J.R.M. and Feely, M. (1988). Tolerance to the anticonvulsant effect of benzodiazepines. *Trends Pharmacolog Sci* **91**, 361–366.

Haigh, J.R.M., Gent, J.P., Garratt, J.C., Pullar, T. and Feely, M. (1988). Disappointing results of increasing benzodiazepine dose after the development of anticonvulsant tolerance. *J Neurol Neurosurg Psychiatry* **51**, 1008–1009.

Heller, A.J., Ring, H.A. and Reynolds, E.H. (1988). Factors relating to a dramatic response to clobazam in refractory epilepsy. *Epilepsy Res* **2**, 276–280.

Hindmarch, I. (1995). The psychopharmacology of clobazam. *Hum Psychopharmacol* **10** (suppl. 1), S15–S25.

Impagnatiello, F., Pesold, C., Longone, P. *et al.* (1996). Modifications of gamma-aminobutyric acid A receptor subunit expression in rat neocortex during tolerance to diazepam. *Mol Pharmacol* **49**, 822–831.

Itier, V., Granger, P., Perrault, G., Depoortere, H., Scatton, B. and Avenet, P. (1996). Protracted treatment with diazepam reduces benzodiazepine 1 receptor-mediated potentiation of gama-aminobutyric acid-induced currents in dissociated rat hippocampal neurons. *J Pharmacol Exp Ther* **279**, 1092–1099.

Loscher, W., Rundfeldt, C., Honack, D. and Ebert, U. (1996). Long-term studies on anticonvulsant tolerance and withdrawal characteristics of benzodiazepine receptor ligands in different seizure models in mice. I. Comparison of diazepam, clonazepam and abecarnil. *J Pharmarcol Exp Ther* **279**, 561–572.

Malizia, A.L. and Nutt, D.J. (1995). Psychopharmacology of benzodiazepines—an update. *Hum Psychopharmacol* **10** (suppl. 1), S1–S14.

Munn, R. and Farrell, K. (1993). Open study of clobazam in refractory epilepsy. *Pediatr Neurol* **9**, 465–469.

Pesold, C., Caruncho, H.J., Impagnatiello, F. *et al.* (1997). Tolerance to diazepam and changes in GABAA receptor subunit expression in rat neocortical areas. *Neuroscience* **79**, 477–487.

Ramsey-Williams, V.A. and Carter, D.B. (1996). Chronic triazolam and its withdrawal alters GABAA receptor subunit mRNA levels: an *in situ* hybridization study. *Brain Res Mol Brain Res* **43**, 132–140.

Reddy, D.S. and Kulkarni, S.K. (1997). Neurosteroid co-administration prevents development of tolerance and augments recovery from benzodiazepine withdrawal anxiety and hyperactivity in mice. *Methods Find Exp Clin Pharmacol* **19**, 395–405.

Remy, C. (1994). Clobazam in the treatment of epilepsy–a review of the literature. *Epilepsia* **35** (suppl 5), S88–S91.

Robertson M.M. (1986). Current status of the 1,4– and 1,5–benzodiazepines in the treatment of epilepsy: the place of clobazam. *Epilepsia* **27** (suppl 1) S27–S41.

Robertson, M.M. (1995). The place of clobazam in the treatment of epilepsy: an update. *Hum Psychopharmacol* **10** (suppl 1), S43–S63.

Rosenberg, H.C., Tietz, E.I. and Chiu, T.H. (1989). Tolerance to anticonvulsant effects of diazepam, clonazepam and clobazam in amygdala-kindled rats. *Epilepsia* **30**, 276–285.

Rundfeldt, C., Wlaz, P., Honack, D. and Loscher, W. (1995). Anticonvulsant tolerance and withdrawal characteristics of benzodiazepine receptor ligands in different seizure models in mice. Comparison of diazepam, betazenil and abecarnil. *J Pharmacol Exp Ther* **275**, 693–702.

Savic, I., Widen, L. and Stone-Elander, S. (1991). Feasibility of reversing benzodiazipine tolerance with flumazenil. *Lancet* **337**, 133–137.

Schmidt, D. (1994). Clobazam for treatment of intractable epilepsy: a critical assessment. *Epilepsia* **35** (suppl 5), S88–S91.

Shorvon, S.D. (1995). Benzodiazepines: clobazam. In: Levy, R.H., Mattson, R.H. and Meldrum, B.S. (Eds), *Antiepileptic Drugs (4th edn)*. Raven Press, New York, 763–778.

Shrader, R.I. and Greenblatt, D.J. (1993). Use of benzodiazepines in anxiety disorders. *N Engl J Med* **328**, 1398–1405.

Singh, A., Guberman, A.H. and Boisvert, D. (1995). Clobazam in long-term epilepsy treatment: sustained responders versus those developing tolerance. *Epilepsia* **36**, 798–803.

Suzuki, Y., Nagai, T. and Okada, S. (1998). Influence of co-administered antiepileptic drugs on nitrazepam tolerance in mice. *No. To. Hattatsu* **30**, 517–522.

Tietz, E.I., Huang, X., Weng, X., Rosenberg, H.C. and Chiu, T.H. (1993). Expression of alpha 1, alpha 5, and gamma 2 GABAA receptor subunit mRNAs measured in situ in rat hippocampus and cortex following chronic flurazepam administration. *J Mol Neurosci* **4**, 277–292.

Tondi, M., Carboni, F., Deriv, A., Manca, S. and Mastropaolo, C. (1987). Intermittent therapy with clobazam for simple febrile convulsions. *Dev Med Child Neurol* **29**, 830–831.

Wildin, J.D. and Pleuvry, B.J. (1992). Tolerance to the anticonvulsant effects of clobazam in mice. *Neuropharmacol* **31**, 129–135.

Zhao, T.J., Chiu, T.H. and Rosenberg, H.C. (1994). Decreased expression of gamma-aminobutyric acid type A/benzodiazepine receptor beta subunit mRNA in brain of flurazepam-tolerant rats. *J Mol Neurosci* **5**, 181–192.

10

Intermittent Use of Benzodiazepines in Epilepsy

MORGAN FEELY

Clinical Pharmacology Unit, University of Leeds and Department of Medicine, Leeds General Infirmary, Leeds, UK

INTRODUCTION

Benzodiazepines, particularly clobazam, may have a useful role as intermittent adjunctive treatment in the management of epilepsy. Clinicians who use clobazam in this way are taking advantage of the useful properties of this drug while recognizing that the existence of a tolerance phenomenon limits its role in long-term treatment. Among the benzodiazepines that have been employed in the treatment of epilepsy, clobazam probably possesses the best balance of efficacy, tolerability and pharmacokinetic parameters to make it a useful inter-mittent oral treatment in chronic epilepsy. Many of the ways it can be usefully employed will be described, using brief patient histories in some instances.

Although the author has spent some time, together with colleagues, exploring ways of minimizing or circumventing the benzodiazepine tolerance phenomenon in epilepsy, it should be pointed out that tolerance is not an 'all or none' phenomenon and that in some patients benzodiazepines, includ-ing clobazam, may have a valuable persisting effect where they are used continuously over many years. Finally, while the issue of benzodiazepine tolerance is the subject of Chapter 9, and while it is preferable to avoid dupli-cation, it is neither logical nor possible to separate completely the topics of tolerance and intermittent benzodiazepine use.

OBSERVATIONS ON ANTICONVULSANT TOLERANCE IN EXPERIMENTAL MODELS RELEVANT TO INTERMITTENT USE IN HUMANS WITH EPILEPSY

During the 1980s, several groups developed animal models in order to characterize tolerance to the anticonvulsant effect of benzodiazepines and/or in order to compare different benzodiazepines in this respect. In general, the results of these experiments are highly consistent with regard to the extent and rate of tolerance development where the same benzodiazepines have been compared in different models. Also, in general, these observations on benzodiazepine tolerance in animal models are consistent with clinical observations on the problem of tolerance when patients with epilepsy are treated with benzodiazepines. In summary (Haigh and Feely, 1988), it can be said that studies on tolerance to the anticonvulsant effect of benzodiazepines in animal models reveal:

- a partial tolerance that evolves gradually during repeated treatment
- relatively rapid recovery of acute/initial activity on cessation of treatment.
- differences between benzodiazepines with regard to the rate and extent of tolerance development
- consistency between the results from different models (and different investigators) when the same drugs have been compared in more than one model.

In groups of laboratory animals bred from a single strain to be as homogeneous as possible, and with a test sufficiently sensitive to show even modest losses in drug effect, individual animals within a test group differ very little with regard to the extent of loss of drug activity during repeated dosing. Not only are patients with epilepsy much more heterogeneous in respect of reasons for having seizures and genetic influences on drug metabolism for example, but there is no yardstick for measuring loss of drug effect until (spontaneous) seizures recur. Given the extensive interindividual variation in the severity of epilepsy and the factors that trigger seizures in humans, there is every reason to expect substantial differences between individuals regarding how much of the drug effect needs to be lost (time elapses) before seizures recur during continued treatment with a benzodiazepine. Indeed, in the case of a tolerance that evolves gradually but appears to be incomplete, it might be expected that clinical tolerance (the recurrence of spontaneous seizures) would not be seen at all in some individuals. This in fact is what is seen in clinical practice when a benzodiazepine such as clobazam is used continuously to treat patients for a period of time. There is evidence of tolerance in most individuals: it can be seen to be a partial tolerance (only) in some and in a few individuals (presumably because the residual drug effect is still sufficient to protect them) seizures do not recur.

Figure 1 represents a schematic model designed to illustrate how in a heterogeneous population, such as humans with epilepsy, gradually evolving (partial) tolerance to a benzodiazepine will result in an anticonvulsant effect which varies substantially in duration (clinical usefulness) in different individuals. It follows from this that the clinical appropriateness/usefulness of intermittent treatment will depend on the individual.

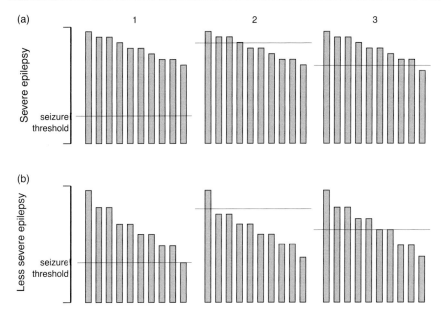

Figure 1 Illustration (schematic) of how achievement and/or maintenance of the therapeutic effect may depend on the individual patient when using a benzodiazepine (BDZ) such as clobazam in the treatment of epilepsy. Before treatment (1, a and b), all of the patients (each represented by a vertical bar to indicate the severity of processes giving rise to their seizures) are having seizures. With treatment (2, a and b), the seizure threshold is raised and many patients stop having seizures; more among the group with less severe epilepsy (2b) than among those with severe epilepsy (2a). When/if a substantial degree of tolerance develops (3, a and b) and the seizure threshold falls back towards (but not to) baseline, most, but not all, of the patients with severe epilepsy (3a) will start having seizures again, while among those with less severe epilepsy (3b) a larger proportion will remain seizure-free.

For patients, such as the one illustrated in Figure 2, where relapse during benzodiazepine treatment does not occur for many months, the concept of developing a strategy of alternating drug treatments is, in theory at least, a very attractive one. Although many observations in animal models (Gent *et al.*, 1998) and humans suggest that because of cross-tolerance the alternate treatment cannot be another benzodiazepine, at least one group (Barcs and Halasz, 1996) have reported an absence of cross-tolerance between two benzodiazepines, clonazepam and clobazam, in patients with epilepsy. As yet, a suitable alternative, for example a drug from another group where there is also good tolerability but where a tolerance phenomenon limits clinical utility, has yet to be identified. Nonetheless, given the usefulness of clobazam in the short/intermediate-term, and the fairly large proportion of patients

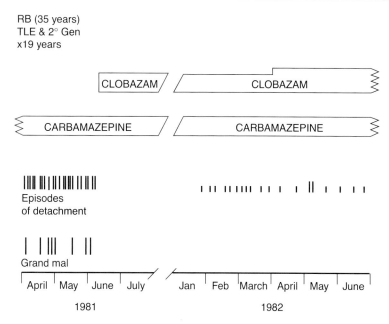

Figure 2 The type of case where tolerance to the antiepileptic effect of a benzodi-azepine, clobazam, is not seen for many months. In cases such as this, alternating treatments, using a drug from another group to cover 'holidays' from clobazam (or another benzodiazepine), might be a successful strategy (see text).

with refractory epilepsy who do not respond satisfactorily to any of the 'new' drugs, this concept remains an attractive one. With regard to the choice of benzodiazepine for this purpose, it should be acknowledged that while clonazepam may be more 'sedative' than clobazam, in animal models it exhibits less tolerance which develops less quickly (Haigh and Feely, 1988). The active metabolite of clobazam, N-desmethylclobazam, also exhibits less tolerance in an animal model and in a limited study in patients with epilepsy appeared to be as or more effective compared with clobazam, and with very good tolerability (Haigh et al., 1987).

In an individual where the loss of effect during repeated use results in the return of frequent seizures within a matter of weeks (or even days), the idea of alternating a benzodiazepine with some other antiepileptic drug would seem unlikely to prove feasible. Nonetheless, employing a benzodiazepine intermittently, as short-term adjunctive treatment, can still be very useful, particularly in cases where there are predictable exacerbations, as in catamenial epilepsy, or in patients where seizures tend to occur in clusters (often with several weeks of freedom from seizures in between).

INTERMITTENT SHORT-TERM USE OF BENZODIAZEPINES IN PATIENTS WITH EPILEPSY

Intermittent clobazam for catamenial epilepsy

In the early 1980s, Feely and colleagues (1982) described the use of catamenial epilepsy (exacerbations of epilepsy around menstruation) as a model in which to evaluate the antiepileptic effect of a benzodiazepine, clobazam, compared with placebo, in a cross-over study. Initially, by giving the trial treatment(s) as short-term adjunctive therapy at a time when the patients virtually always had clusters of seizures, it was possible to compare the antiepileptic effect of the two treatments, 'separated' from the tolerance issue. The same investigators (Feely and Gibson, 1984) were able to follow many of the same patients while they received intermittent clobazam treatment around menstruation for a duration ranging from a couple of months to three and a half years, and demonstrated both that this form of treatment was useful for many patients and that tolerance could be avoided by intermittent treatment (Table 1). This 'experiment' in patients seems to have antedated any studies formally evaluating intermittent benzodiazepine use in animal models, where intermittent treatment with clonazepam appears to prevent anticonvulsant tolerance in mice (Suzuki et al., 1993).

Table 1. Results of intermittent treatment with clobazam in catamenial epilepsy.

Case no.	Duration and outcome of treatment	Seizures while taking clobazam	Increase in seizures between periods
1	5 months (D)	20[a] (per period)	No
2	12 months (B)	None	No
3	3.5 years (A)	None	No
4	15 months (B)	1 (total)	No
5	6 months (X)	None	No
6	12 months (X)	None	Yes
7	2 months (E)	6 on 10 mg None on 20 mg	No
8	4 months (C)	None	Yes
9	3 years (A)	None	No
10	12 months (X)	1 (total)	No
11	13 months (X)	None	No
12	3 years (A)	None	No
13	12 months (C)	None	Yes

Outcome of long-term treatment: (A) still using clobazam;
(B) successful treatment until pregnancy; (C) clobazam stopped when seizures between periods increased; (D) treatment changed because of poor overall control; (E) clobazam stopped because of sedative effects; (X) regarded as not clearly determined due to insufficient follow-up.
[a] Approximately 40% of pretreatment number.
Source: From Feely and Gibson, 1984.

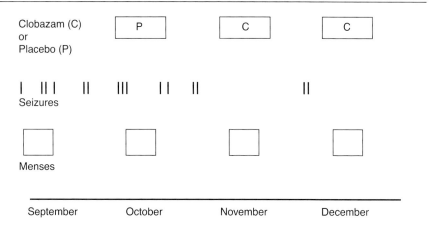

Figure 3 The use of clobazam in a typical patient with catamenial epilepsy, receiving a placebo for one period and then clobazam for two periods. While this does not render the patient, who also has seizures at other times (e.g. mid-cycle), seizure-free, it provides both freedom from the 'bad patches' around menstruation and an overall reduction in seizures (about 50% in this example).

Figure 3 illustrates the reduction in seizures achieved in a typical case, initially in comparison with a period on placebo. In those (uncommon) cases where patients only have seizures around menstruation, this form of treatment may render a patient seizure-free, or virtually seizure-free. The case history that follows represents an example of the possible long-term benefit with this form of treatment.

Case history

Patricia (one of the patients designated as outcome 'B' in Table 1) had meningitis at 5 months old and developed temporal lobe epilepsy at the age of 7 years. Despite trying a number of different drugs (primidone, carbamazepine, valproate) her seizures were never well controlled and at the age of 22 years she was still having frequent seizures (usually somewhere between five and 12 per month). Most of these attacks were compound forms of partial seizures and there were exacerbations during the few days before menstruation began in virtually every menstrual cycle. Because of this she was commenced on clobazam (20 mg per day for 10 days) as adjunctive treatment around menstruation, in addition to her regular medication (carbamazepine, primidone). With 'time out' for two pregnancies she has now been using that form of adjunctive treatment around menstruation for 18 years. Overall, it has reduced her seizures by approximately 50%. She still tends to have some attacks in most months; these occur particularly mid-cycle (possibly at ovulation). Her periods tend to be somewhat irregular and when a period (and seizures related to same) commences sooner than expected she may have one or two seizures before, or on the first day of, the clobazam therapy. Recently, two periods occurred closer together than usual and she had only been off the clobazam for 8 days before she started another course. She then noticed that after 5 or 6 days of clobazam therapy she began to get 'warnings'. With these exceptions she has normally been seizure-free around menstruation while using clobazam and, where attempts to change her definitive treatment (in the hope of achieving final control) were not successful, this treatment has provided considerable benefit, with a marked improvement in her quality of life.

Intermittent benzodiazepine therapy for the prevention or treatment of seizures occurring in clusters in situations other than catamenial epilepsy

Many patients with intractable epilepsy can have severe seizures at any time. In the case of some patients whose epilepsy is not adequately controlled, with established treatments these exacerbations of epilepsy make take the form of clusters of seizures. While these may not be as predictable as the exacerbations seen in cases of catamenial epilepsy, in some patients there may be known precipitating factors, such as travel or excitement/stress related to a 'big event'. Short courses of a benzodiazepine, usually clobazam, as adjunctive treatment may be useful in one of two ways.

1. In the patient with severe epilepsy who may have sporadic but severe seizures at any time, a short course of clobazam can be used *preventively* to 'cover' important events. Usually this is some family occasion (wedding, party), an examination, an interview, a business trip or a holiday; circumstances in which severe seizures would be particularly inconvenient, especially if they gave rise to the patient being taken to hospital. Clobazam, given intermittently, has also been used to cover busulphan chemotherapy (Schwarer *et al.*, 1995) and as prophylaxis/treatment of seizures during febrile episodes in children (Manreza *et al.*, 1997).

Case history: clobazam prophylaxis to cover holidays

Jane, now in her twenties, has had intractable epilepsy since early childhood and despite conventional therapy she still has frequent exacerbations, which often take the form of clusters of two or three grand mal seizures. She also has learning difficulties and is resident in a hostel. Once or twice each year the residents go away together for a brief holiday under the supervision of hostel staff. After Jane had to be taken to hospital because of seizures during two successive holidays, it was decided to cover holidays with a short course (about 10 days) of clobazam, starting two or three days before departure. Since this measure was instituted there have been several further holidays – all without problems.

2. Oral clobazam can also be used to *treat* clusters of seizures/serial attacks, particularly when these are partial seizures. Other benzodiazepines that may be given by other routes to achieve the same end include diazepam (rectal) and midazolam (nasal/buccal). At a certain point, the use of rectal diazepam (given, for example, at home by a family member) to treat severe seizures overlaps with the management of status epilepticus, which is the subject of Chapter 7. However, clobazam (by mouth) can be given to patients in *non-convulsive* status and in suitable patients represents an attractive treatment option; this has been reported to work in cases of partial status where other treatments, including other benzodiazepines, have failed (Corman *et al.*, 1998).

Case history: oral clobazam for treating attacks in clusters

David, who was born in 1932, has had intractable epilepsy since the age of 9 years, with complex partial (temporal lobe) and grand mal seizures. He also has mild learning difficulties. In the early 1980s, 'fine tuning' of his phenytoin dose produced much improved, but still incomplete, seizure control. Subsequently, an attempt to replace phenytoin with lamotrigine failed and he now takes a slightly reduced dose of phenytoin together with lamotrigine. He lives alone, but a brother and his family live very close by and keep an eye on him. From time to time, on average perhaps every 4–6 months, he develops clusters of serial complex partial seizures. These often start early in the day and previously he would be 'out of it' for the whole day. His brother would put him to bed but on occasions the episodes culminated with grand mal seizures, sometimes leading to admission to hospital. For some years his brother has been giving him a single oral (10 or 20 mg) dose of clobazam when he observes the onset of partial seizures. Typically, the episode is now terminated within an hour or two, and David can go about his normal activities later in the day with only rare hospital admission required. Interestingly, on a recent (atypical) occasion when one cluster followed within a week of the last one, it seemed that the clobazam was of little effect and David again spent a night in hospital.

Why clobazam for single-dose or short-term use?

Many benzodiazepines have been used/evaluated in epilepsy, but clobazam appears to be the best oral drug for these short-term applications. For these purposes a drug needs good initial tolerability, rapid onset of effect and few relevant/significant interactions. For example, few patients would be able to tolerate full therapeutic doses of clonazepam (also available as an oral treatment; probably less subject to tolerance) on the first day of treatment. While clobazam, in common with other benzodiazepines, may (rarely) inhibit phenytoin metabolism (Zifkin *et al.*, 1991), this is very unlikely to be of clinical significance when clobazam is only added to the regimen for between 1 and 10 days. Above all, in acute use, oral clobazam (as a single dose or in short courses) has been shown by experience to have a very satisfactory therapeutic index (balance of efficacy and toxicity).

REFERENCES

Barcs, G. and Halasz, P. (1996). Effectiveness and tolerance of clobazam in temporal lobe epilepsy. *Acta Neurol Scand* **93**, 88–93.

Corman, C., Guberman, A. and Benavente, O. (1998). Clobazam in partial status epilepticus. *Seizure* **7**, 243–247.

Feely, M. and Gibson, J. (1984). Intermittent clobazam for catamenial epilepsy: tolerance avoided. *J Neurol Neurosurg Psychiatry* **47**, 1279–1282.

Feely, M., Calvert, R. and Gibson, J. (1982). Clobazam in catamenial epilepsy: a model for evaluating anticonvulsants. *Lancet* **ii**, 71–73.

Gent, J.P., Bentley, M., Feely, M. and Haigh, J.R.M. (1998). Benzodiazepine cross tolerance in mice extends to sodium valproate. *Eur J Pharmacol* **12**, 89–15.

Haigh, J.R.M. and Feely, N.Y. (1988). Tolerance to the anticonvulsant effect of benzodiazepines. *Trends Pharmacol Sci* **9**, 361–366.

Haigh, J.R.M., Pullar, T., Gent, J.P., Dailley, C. and Feely, M. (1987). *N*-desmethylclobazam: a possible alternative to clobazam in the treatment of refractory epilepsy? *Br J Clin Pharmacol* **23**, 213–218.

Manreza, M., Gherpelli, J.L., Machado-Haertel, L.R., Pedreira, C.C., Heise, C.O. and Diament, A. (1997). Treatment of febrile seizures with intermittent clobazam. *Arq Neuropsiquiatr* **55**, 757–761.

Schwarer, A.P., Opat, S.S., Watson, A.L. and Cole-Sinclair, M.F. (1995). Clobazam for seizure prophylaxis during busulfan chemotherapy. *Lancet* **346**, 1238.

Suzuki, Y., Edge, J., Mimaki, T. and Watson, P. (1993). Intermittent clonazepam treatment prevents anticonvulsant tolerance in mice. *Epilepsy Res* **15**, 15–20.

Zifkin, B., Sherwin, A. and Andermann, F. (1991). Phenytoin toxicity due to interaction with clobazam. *Neurology* **41**, 313–314.

Benzodiazepines
Edited by Michael R. Trimble and Ian Hindmarch
© 2000 Wrightson Biomedical Publishing Ltd

11

Benzodiazepines in the Treatment of Movement Disorders related to Epilepsy

KAILASH P. BHATIA

*Department of Clinical Neurology, Institute of Neurology,
University College London, London, UK*

INTRODUCTION

Movement disorders are traditionally thought to be extrapyramidal disorders caused by basal ganglia dysfunction. However, although this is true in the broad sense it is well known that lesions or dysfunction of other areas of the central or even the peripheral nervous system can cause movement disorders. Movement disorders are broadly divided into two groups: disorders causing diminished (or less than normal) movements, for example Parkinson's disease; and disorders with excessive abnormal involuntary movements or dyskinesias (Table 1).

Benzodiazepines, particularly clonazepam or diazepam, have been found to be very useful for a variety of movement disorders, particularly in patients with different dyskinesias, manifesting mainly as jerks or sustained spasms (Tables 2 and 3). Historically, the interest in benzodiazepines for treating

Table 1. Classification of movement disorders.

Hypokinetic (less than normal movements)
• Parkinson's disease
• Parkinsonian syndromes

Hyperkinetic (involuntary movements)
• Tremor
• Chorea
• Tics
• Myoclonus
• Startle syndromes
• Dystonia

Table 2. Movement disorders manifesting jerks or spasms for which
benzodiazepines may be useful.

Jerks	Spasms
Myoclonus	Dystonia
Tics	Myoclonic dystonia
Startle syndromes	Stiff-man syndrome
Restless legs	Tonic spasms of multiple sclerosis
Paroxysmal movement disorders	

Table 3. Other dyskinetic movement disorders for which benzodiazepines
(particularly clonazepam) can be useful.

Tremor (especially jerky tremors)
Palatal tremor (myoclonus)
Orthostatic tremor
Belly dancers' dyskinesia
Tardive dyskinesias
Levodopa-induced dyskinesia in Parkinson's disease

Table 4. Movement disorders related to epilepsy.

Myoclonic disorders
Startle syndromes
Paroxysmal dyskinesias
• Paroxysmal kinesigenic choreoathetosis
• Paroxysmal non-kinesigenic choreoathetosis
• Hypnogenic (nocturnal) dyskinesia
• Frontal lobe seizures and other partial epilepsies

different movement disorders probably started when clonazepam was found
to be particularly useful in treating post-anoxic myoclonus (Jenner *et al.*,
1986). Clonazepam is a 1,4- benzodiazepine structurally related to diazepam
and nitrazepam. It is known to inhibit pentylenetetrazole-induced seizures.
It interacts with benzodiazepine brain receptors facilitating gamma-aminobutyric acid (GABA)ergic transmission (and probably also dopamine, 5-
hydroxytryptamine, and noradrenergic systems).

Jenner and colleagues (1986) showed that clonazepam was better for treating post-anoxic myoclonus compared with diazepam. It is interesting to note
that clonazepam appears to be the favoured benzodiazepine in the
movement disorder literature to treat all forms of disorders, with little
mention of other benzodiazepines apart from diazepam.

This chapter will concentrate on the use of benzodiazepines in movement
disorders that are thought be (directly or indirectly) related to epilepsy.

These comprise three main groups (Table 4): the myoclonic disorders, startle syndromes, and some of the paroxysmal movement disorders.

THE MYOCLONIC DISORDERS

Myoclonus can be defined as an abrupt and brief muscle jerk. Myoclonic jerks can be classified depending on the origin of the discharge in the nervous system. *Segmental* myoclonus is due to an abnormal discharge from the spinal cord or brainstem usually affecting one body part alone; *reticular* myoclonus is due to discharges in the brainstem; and *cortical* myoclonus, which can cause reflex (touch, muscle stretch, or other stimulus-induced) jerks, action-induced myoclonus or spontaneous jerks (including epilepsia partialis continua). Electrophysiological techniques can help in identifying the origin of the discharge and this has therapeutic implications because benzo-diazepines (clonazepam) seem more effective in cortical compared with sub-cortical myoclonus.

Cortical myoclonus

Cortical myoclonus is distinguished by the presence of spike discharges on electroencephalogram (EEG) time-locked to the electromyogram (EMG) burst on back-averaging and enlarged somatosensory-evoked responses. Both idiopathic (e.g. essential myoclonus) and symptomatic conditions, including cerebral anoxia and a variety of progressive neurodegenerative disorders (Table 5), can cause cortical myoclonus.

Brainstem reticular myoclonus

This is relatively rare. Reticular myoclonus can cause generalized spontaneous and reflex jerks, and recordings can demonstrate that muscles are recruited in sequence up the brainstem and down the spinal cord. Like cortical myoclonus, there are numerous causes of brainstem reticular myoclonus, the most common being post-anoxic myoclonus, brainstem encephalitis and uraemia. It should be noted that reticular myoclonus may co-exist with cortical myoclonus.

Propriospinal myoclonus

This manifests as axial flexion jerks involving the trunk, neck and hip muscles. These manifest spontaneously usually when the patient is lying flat or standing, or can be precipitated by somaesthetic stimuli (Brown *et al.*, 1991). Spinal generators recruit muscles up and down the spinal cord via long propriospinal pathways (Brown *et al.*, 1991). Spinal cord trauma, usually cervical, is the cause in nearly 50% of cases.

Table 5. Aetiological classification of cortical myoclonus.

Symptomatic myoclonus
Storage disorders
- Lafora body disease
- Ceroid-lipofuscinosis
- Sialidosis
Mitochondrial disorders
Spinocerebellar degenerations
- Baltic myoclonus (Unverricht–Lundborg disease)
- Ataxia telangiectasia
Basal ganglia degenerations
- Wilson's disease
- Huntington's disease
- Dentato-rubro-pallidoluysian atrophy
- Corticobasal degeneration
- Multiple system atrophy
- Progressive supranuclear palsy
Dementias
- Prion diseases
- Alzheimer's disease
Malabsorption syndromes
- Whipple's disease
- Coeliac disease
Viral encephalopathies
Metabolic encephalopathies
- Hepatic failure
- Renal failure
Toxic encephalopathies
- Bismuth
- Heavy metals
Physical encephalopathies
- Post anoxic (Lance Adams syndrome)
- Post head injury

Physiological myoclonus
- Sleep jerks
- Hiccoughs

Essential myoclonus

Epileptic myoclonus (seizures predominate, no encephalopathy)
Fragments of epilepsy
- Isolated epileptic myoclonic jerks
- Epilepsia partialis continua
- Photosensitive myoclonus
- Myoclonic absences in petit mal
Childhood myoclonic epilepsies

Spinal segmental myoclonus

This produces rhythmic jerking confined to one or two contiguous myotomes. It can be caused by a variety of spinal pathologies, which essentially lead to isolation of the spinal motoneurons from inhibitory influences. Intrinsic and extrinsic malignancies, syringomyelia and inflammatory conditions are common causes.

THE ROLE OF BENZODIAZEPINES IN THE TREATMENT OF MYOCLONUS

The treatment of different forms of myoclonus has been reviewed recently by Brown (1995). For cortical myoclonus, the first choice is valproate or clonazepam. Piracetam can be added to these and primidone or phenobarbitone are other options. The first line of treatment for brainstem reticular myoclonus is also valproate or clonazepam. Clonazepam is found to be helpful in nearly 50% of cases with propriospinal myoclonus.

The treatment of segmental spinal myoclonus is that of the underlying cause if that is possible. For symptomatic treatment, clonazepam is the drug of choice and in dosages up to 6 mg a day may diminish or abolish the myoclonus (Hoehn and Cherrington, 1977; Jankovic and Pardo, 1986). Diazepam, in dosages up to 30 mg daily (Hopkins and Michael, 1974), carbamazepine and tetrabenazine are other choices (Jankovic and Pardo, 1986).

In summary, clonazepam is extremely useful in all types of myoclonic disorders, in particular for cortical myoclonus. However, it has been shown that combination therapy consisting of sodium valproate, clonazepam and piracetam improves action myoclonus of cortical origin better than when any of these drugs were used alone (Obeso et al., 1989).

THE STARTLE SYNDROMES

Hyperekplexia

There is an inherited autosomal dominant disorder also called startle disease. It is characterized by exaggerated startle reactions to unexpected stimuli, particularly auditory. Startle reactions are marked by a short period of generalized stiffness (tonic spasm) during which voluntary movements are impossible. Consciousness is preserved. In addition, hypertonicity is often present, which is first noticed at birth with the child having stiff legs, a flexed posture and clenching of the fists. The stiffness usually gradually diminishes over the first years of life, although in some it may be present throughout life often exacerbated by cold and other factors.

The genetic defect of hereditary hyperekplexia has been identified as a point mutation in the $\alpha1$ subunit of the glycine receptor on chromosome 5q33 (Shiang et al.,1993; 1995; Tijssen et al., 1995). Sporadic cases that do not carry the glycine receptor mutations have also been described (Shiang et al., 1995).

On electrophysiologeal investigation, brainstem pathways have been impli-
cated with the suggestion that there was dysfunction of the rhombomesen-
cephalic reticular formation resulting in an abnormal release of the startle
pathways. The pattern of muscle recruitment is similar to reticular reflex
myoclonus except that the efferent conduction down the spinal cord is slower
(Brown *et al.*, 1990). There is also a suggestion of cerebral hyperexcitability
in hyperekplexia, with EEG spikes in some cases (Andermann *et al.*, 1980).

Several drugs have been tried in hyperekplexia. In the hereditary form,
various benzodiazepines, such as diazepam, chlordiazepoxide, clonazepam
(Brown *et al.*, 1991), and antiepileptics, such as carbamazepine and phenytoin (Brown *et al.*, 1991), were incidentally found to be successful. In sporadic
cases, diazepam, 5-hydroxytryptophan, piracetam, vigabatrin and phenobarbitone were all reported to be effective.

However, clonazepam appears to be consistently beneficial for both the
hereditary and sporadic varieties of hyperekplexia and is the drug of choice.
Many authors have reported that clonazepam reduces the frequency and
magnitude of the startle response and reduces the frequency of falls due to
transient stiffness. The beneficial effects of clonazepam are probably related
to its GABA potentiating effect. The interaction between the two major
spinal inhibitory systems glycine and GABA are not fully understood. Both
are ligand gated ion channel receptors sharing considerable structural and
sequence homology. It is questionable whether the point mutation in the
glycine subunit in hereditary hyperekplexia causes an increase in the responsiveness to GABA (and therefore the benefit from clonazepam), but this has
not been substantiated. In an interesting study to test whether or not the effect
of clonazepam is due to an increase in GABA activity, Tijssen and colleagues
(1997), in a double-blind, cross-over study compared clonazepam with vigabatrin (a specific inhibitor of GABA-transaminase) using objective measures of
motor startle responses and scores of stiffness and drowsiness in four patients
with hereditary hyperekplexia. Clonazepam but not vigabatrin significantly
reduced the magnitude of the motor startle response in these patients. The
authors postulated that the effect may not be based on the indirect increase
in GABA, but may be due to the direct effect of clonazepam on the modified
$\alpha 1$ subunit of the glycine receptor (Tijssen *et al.*, 1997).

Startle epilepsy

Startle epilepsy is characterized by epileptic seizures triggered by sudden
unexpected startle produced by any stimulus (auditory being the most effective). Startle epilepsy has been described in the setting of severe brain
damage owing to a variety of disorders, including anoxic perinatal
encephalopathy, Lennox–Gastaut syndrome, West's syndrome and Down's
syndrome. Saenz-Lope and colleagues (1984a) divided their patients into two

groups: those with hemiparesis due to hemispheric lesions and normal background EEG; and those with more severe diffuse brain damage, marked intellectual impairment, generalized seizures (not related to startle) and background EEG abnormalities.

Treatment of startle epilepsy is difficult. Saenz-Lope and colleagues (1984b) found carbamazepine to be useful in their patients with the hemiparetic form. For the generalized form, valproic acid, carbamazepine and clonazepam were found to be beneficial, including two patients with the Lennox–Gastaut syndrome. Tinuper and colleagues (1986) reported the beneficial effect of clobazam in 8 of 13 patients who were previously on an ineffective regime.

PAROXYSMAL MOVEMENT DISORDERS AS A MANIFESTATION OF EPILEPSY

Paroxysmal movement disorders are defined as abnormal involuntary movements occurring episodically with no abnormality detected interictally. Any form of dyskinetic activity, including chorea, myoclonus, dystonia or a combination, may occur during the episode. Consciousness is not lost. Traditionally, the paroxysmal dyskinesias are classified by the trigger and duration of the attack (Lance, 1977; Demirkirin and Jankovic, 1995) and whether the condition is idiopathic (often familial) or due to a symptomatic cause.

In paroxysmal kinesigenic choreoathetosis (PKC), the attacks are precipitated by sudden movement (i.e. kinesigenic), are brief in duration (less than 5 minutes), frequent and respond well to anticonvulsants (Houser *et al.*, 1999). On the other hand, in paroxysmal dystonic choreoathetosis (PDC) the attacks are of long duration (many hours) and are precipitated by coffee, alcohol and fatigue but not sudden movement (Demirkirin and Jankovic, 1995). An intermediate form is paroxysmal exercise-induced dyskinesia (PED) in which the attacks occur on prolonged exercise, usually walking or swimming, and last a few minutes to an hour (Lance, 1977). Lastly, in paroxysmal nocturnal (hypogenic) dyskinesia, the attacks occur at night during sleep.

There remains much controversy regarding the pathophysiology of these disorders. Many authors regard PKC as a form of reflex epilepsy involving the basal ganglia (Lishman *et al.*, 1962; Falconer *et al.*, 1963) because of the brevity of episodes and excellent response to anticonvulsants. A subcortical focus is likely because of the absence of seizure discharges on EEG, the absence of evolution of the attacks into generalized or focal convulsions, and the lack of an associated loss of consciousness or amnesia. In support of this is a patient described by Falconer and colleagues (1963) whose movement-induced seizures stopped after excision of a cortical scar from the left supplementary motor cortex. Also, with depth electrode recordings in one patient with PKC, Lombroso (1995) showed that during an attack discharges arose in the supplementary motor area and spread to the basal ganglia. It is now recognized that epilepsy can mimic or produce various movement disorders if motor phenomena predominate in the absence of the well-recognized seizure pattern, i.e. loss of awareness, generalized tonic-clonic activity and a normal scalp EEG (Fish and Marsden, 1994).

This problem has been exemplified by frontal lobe epilepsies. These present with bizarre motor attacks sometimes involving all four limbs, without loss of consciousness and with apparently normal interictal and ictal EEGs (Meierkord *et al.*, 1992). Hypnogenic paroxysmal dystonia is now recognized as a form of frontal lobe epilepsy in many cases (Tinuper *et al.*, 1990), and families with this disorder have been described by Scheffer and colleagues (1995) under the acronym ADNFLE (autosomal dominant frontal lobe epilepsy). The similarities of paroxysmal dyskinesia, particularly PKC to episodic ataxia type 1, which is known to be mutation in the potassium channel gene (Browne *et al.*, 1994), suggest that these disorders (and indeed many epileptic disorders) may be due to defects of ion channels, i.e. channellopathies. In this regard, two PDC families have been linked to chromosome 2q in the vicinity of anion channel genes (Fink *et al.*, 1996; Fouad *et al.*, 1996) and ADNFLE is known to be caused by a mutation of the neuronal acetylcholine receptor gene on chromosome 20q (Philips *et al.*, 1995).

With regard treatment, PKC and ADNFLE respond best to carbamazepine or phenytoin. Patients with PED and PDC do not respond to these anticonvulsants but some patients have had benefit with clonazepam, which should be tried in these cases (Bhatia *et al.*, 1997).

CONCLUSIONS

In conclusion, it is clear that benzodiazepines, particularly clonazepam, have been found to be very effective and useful in the treatment of a variety of movement disorders related to epilepsy, and particularly for cortical myoclonus. However, benzodiazepines are obviously useful for spasms and jerks of other movement disorders (not related to epilepsy), particularly for jerky dystonia. It is interesting to note that clobazam and other newer benzodiazepines do not find favour with movement disorder specialists, and there is a need for comparative studies on the effectiveness of newer agents, such as clobazam versus clonazepam.

REFERENCES

Andermann, F., Keene, D.L., Andermann, E. and Quesney, L.F. (1980). Startle disease or hyperekplexia: further delineation of the syndrome. *Brain* **103**, 985–997.

Bhatia, K.P., Soland, V.L., Bhatt, B.H., Quinn, N.P. and Marsden, C.D. (1997). Paroxysmal exercise-induced dystonia: eight new sporadic cases and a review of the literature. *Mov Disord* **12**, 1007–1012.

Brown, P. (1995). The treatment of myoclonus. *CNS Drugs* **3**, 22–29.

Brown, P., Rothwell, R.C., Thompson, P.D., Britton, T.C., Day, B.L. and Marsden, C.D. (1990). Reticular reflex myoclonus and its relationship to the normal startle reflex in humans. *Neurology* **40** (suppl 1), 386.

Brown, P., Thompson, P.D., Rothwell, J.C., Day, B.L. and Marsden, C.D. (1991). Axial myoclonus of propriospinal origin. *Brain* **114**, 197–214.

Browne, D.L., Gancher, S.T., Nutt, J.G. *et al.* (1994). Episodic ataxia myokimia syndrome is associated with point mutations in the human potassium channel gene, KCNA1. *Nat Genet* **8**, 136–140.

Demirkirin, M. and Jankovic, J. (1995). Paroxysmal dyskinesias: clinical features and classification. *Ann Neurol* **38**, 571–579.

Falconer, M., Driver, M. and Serafetinides, E. (1963). Seizures induced by movement: report of case relieved by operation. *J Neurol Neurosurg Psychiatry* **26**, 300–307.

Fink, J.K., Rainer, S., Wilkowski, J. *et al.* (1996). Paroxysmal dystonic choreoathetosis. Tight linkage to chromosome 2q. *Am J Hum Genet* **59**, 1490–1495.

Fish, D.R. and Marsden, C.D. (1994). Epilepsy masquerading as a movement disorder. In: Marsden, C.D. and Fahn, S. (Eds), *Movement Disorders 3*. Butterworth-Heinemann, Oxford, pp. 346–358.

Fouad, G.T., Sevidei, S., Durcan, S., Bertini, E. and Ptacek, L.J. (1996). A gene for familial dyskinesia (FPD1) maps to chromosome 2q. *Am J Hum Genet* **59**, 135–139.

Hoehn, M.M. and Cherrington, M. (1977). Spinal myoclonus. *Neurology* **27**, 942–946.

Hopkins, A.P. and Michael, W.F. (1974). Spinal myoclonus. *J Neurol Neurosurg Psychiatry* **37**, 1112–1115.

Houser, M., Soland, V., Bhatia, K.P., Quinn, N.P. and Marsden, C.D. (1999). Paroxysmal kinesiginic choreoathetosis—a report of 26 patients. *J Neurol* **246**, 120–126.

Jankovic, J. and Pardo, R. (1986). Segmental myoclonus. *Arch Neurol* **43**, 1025–1031.

Jenner, P., Pratt, J.A. and Marsden, C.D. (1986). Mechanism of action of clonazepam in myoclonus in relation to effects on GABA and 5HT. *Adv Neurol* **43**, 629–643.

Lance, J.W. (1977). Familial paroxysmal dystonic choreoathetosis and its differentiation from related syndromes. *Ann Neurol* **2**, 285–293.

Lishman, W.A., Symonds, C.D., Whitty, C.W. and Wilson, R.G. (1962). Seizures induced by movement. *Brain* **85**, 93–108.

Lombroso, C.T. (1995). Paroxysmal choreoathetosis: an epileptic or non-epileptic disorder? *Ital J Neurol Sci* **16**, 271–277.

Meierkord, H., Fish, D.R., Smith, S.J.M., Scott, C.A., Shorvon, S.D. and Marsden, C.D. (1992). Is nocturnal dystonia a form of frontal lobe epilepsy? *Mov Disord* **7**, 38–42.

Obeso, J.A., Arteida, J., Rothwell, J.C., Day, B., Thompson, P. and Marsden, C.D. (1989). The treatment of severe action myoclonus. *Brain* **112**, 765–777.

Philips, H.A., Scheffer, I.E., Berkovic, S.F., Holloway, G.E., Sutherland, G.R. and Muller, J.C. (1995). Localization of a gene for autosomal dominant nocturnal frontal lobe epilepsy to chromosome 20q 13.2. *Nat Genet* **10**, 117–118.

Saenz-Lope, E., Herranz-Tanarro, F.J., Masdeu, J.C. and Chacon-Pena, J.R. (1984a). Hyperekplexia: a syndrome of pathological startle responses. *Ann Neurol* **15**, 36–41.

Saenz-Lope, E., Herranz, F.J. and Masdeu, J.C. (1984b). Startle epilepsy: a clinical study. *Ann Neurol* **16**, 78–81.

Scheffer, I.E., Bhatia, K.P., Lopes-Cendes, I. *et al*. (1995). Autosomal dominant nocturnal frontal lobe epilepsy. A distinctive clinical disorder. *Brain* **118**, 61–73.

Shiang, R., Ryan, S.G., Zhu, Y. *et al*. (1993). Mutations in the alpha 1 subunit of the inhibitory glycine receptor cause the dominant neurological disorder, hyperekplexia. *Nat Genet* **5**, 351–357.

Shiang, R., Ryan, S.G., Zhen, Z.R. *et al*. (1995). Mutational analysis of familial and sporadic hyperekplexia. *Ann Neurol* **38**, 85–91.

Tijssen, M.A.J., Shiang, R., Deutckom, J. *et al*. (1995). Molecular genetic reevaluation of the Dutch hyperekplexia family. *Arch Neurol* **52**, 578–582.

Tijssen, M.A.J., Shoemaker, H.C., Edelbroek, P.J., Roos, R.A.C., Cohen, A.F. and Van Dijk, J.G. (1997). The effects of clonazepam and vigabatrin in hyperekplexia. *J Neurol Sci* **149**, 63–67.

Tinuper, P., Aguglia, U. and Gastaut, H. (1986). Use of clobazam in certain forms of status epilepticus and in startle-induced epileptic seizures. *Epilepsia* **27** (suppl 1), S18–S26.

Tinuper, P., Cerullo, A., Cirignotti, F., Cortelli, P., Lugaresi, E. and Montagna, P. (1990). Nocturnal paroxysmal dystonia with short lasting attacks: three cases with evidence for an epileptic frontal lobe origin of seizures. *Epilepsia* **31**, 549–556.

Benzodiazepines
Edited by Michael R. Trimble and Ian Hindmarch
© 2000 Wrightson Biomedical Publishing Ltd

12

Pharmacoeconomics: A Cost-Effectiveness Study of Four Antiepileptic Drugs

CAROLINE E. SELAI, MICHAEL R. TRIMBLE and JAMES LAVETT

Raymond Way Neuropsychiatry Unit, Institute of Neurology, London, UK

INTRODUCTION

In recent years, the costs of medical care in general, and the cost of antiepileptic drugs in particular, have come under close scrutiny (Shorvon, 1997). Whilst approximately 70% of patients are well controlled on monotherapy, with standard antiepileptic drugs, for the remaining 30% of patients polytherapy is considered. Costs rise because combinations of antiepileptic drugs often include the newer compounds and the unit cost of these is much greater than that of the older, more established drugs. Costs of polytherapy are also higher because of increased side effects, additional medical interventions and more extensive drug monitoring. Higher costs might be justified if the newer antiepileptic drugs were more effective than standard agents but the evidence to date does not suggest that they are. A retrospective audit of patients starting on lamotrigine and vigabatrin found that, at 6–8 years follow-up, 86% of those patients still living were no longer taking these add-on drugs (Walker *et al.*, 1996). In another audit, where efficacy was defined as > 50% reduction in seizure frequency, 36% of patients receiving lamotrigine, 29% receiving vigabatrin and 15% receiving gabapentin benefited according to this criterion (McDonnell and Morrow, 1996). A further piece of evidence is the relative cost-effectiveness of the drugs, and formal economic evaluation has now become important.

QUALITY OF LIFE

There is a fundamental tension in the measurement of quality of life (QOL). Since what is deemed important for QOL is acknowledged to be subjective and idiosyncratic, differences being influenced by a variety of personal and cultural factors, an appraisal of QOL should strive to capture the individual's subjectively appraised phenomenological experience. On the other hand, the hallmark of scientific measurements is reliable, 'objective', empirical data collection. QOL researchers have addressed measurement at various stages of this 'subjective/objective' continuum and over one thousand instruments now exist that have been developed taking a variety of approaches to measurement (Hedrick *et al.*, 1996). The two aspects of the qualitative–quantitative continuum have different strengths. It has been suggested that qualitative methods are more valid whilst quantitative methods are more reliable (Mays and Pope, 1996).

The QOL literature advocates a robust and rigorous programme of instrument development and testing, and most QOL measures are developed within the psychometric tradition (McDowell and Newell, 1987; Juniper *et al.*, 1996). Some researchers have argued, however, that since QOL is a uniquely personal perception, most standardized measurements of QOL in the medical literature seem to aim at the wrong target (Gill, 1995). It is argued that QOL can be measured only by determining the opinions of patients and by supplementing (or replacing) the instruments developed by 'experts' (Gill and Feinstein, 1994). Scales developed within the psychometric tradition often omit items important to the beliefs and values of individual patients (Gill, 1995), and the psychometric aim of internal reliability is in conflict with the goals of achieving comprehensiveness and content validity (Brazier and Deverill, 1999). In response to this, a number of 'individualized', patient-driven techniques have been developed whereby the patient can nominate items of importance to him/herself (Guyatt *et al.*, 1987a, b; Geddes *et al.*, 1990; Tugwell *et al.*, 1990; Fraser *et al.*, 1993; O'Boyle *et al.*, 1993; Ruta *et al.*, 1994).

A number of techniques to assess the QOL of patients with epilepsy have been developed within the psychometric tradition (Trimble and Dodson, 1994; Vickrey, 1995; Cramer, 1996). An individualized approach, the Quality of Life Assessment by Construct Analysis (QoLASCA) was developed as a generic tool to assess the QOL of patients with neurological disorders, particularly epilepsy (McGuire, 1991; Kendrick and Trimble, 1994; Kendrick, 1997).

The QoLASCA was derived from the psychological theories and methods Personal Construct Theory and the Repertory Grid Technique (RGT) (Fransella and Bannister, 1977). The full RGT was lengthy and cumbersome and it was deemed desirable to streamline the method. The brief version has been used in a study of patients with epilepsy (Selai and Trimble, 1998), Gilles de la Tourette syndrome (Elstner *et al.*, unpublished results) and dementia (Selai *et al.*, 2000). Preliminary results have shown the revised method to be reliable, valid and more sensitive to post-treatment changes than some other QOL measures. Full psychometric testing is ongoing.

There are strong arguments in favour of a number of approaches to QOL measurement. In practice, the choice of QOL assessment technique depends on the goal of the study and the type of data required, which in turn, will depend upon the use to which the data will be put.

ECONOMIC EVALUATION

There are many types of economic evaluation (Gold *et al.*, 1996; Jefferson *et al.*, 1996; Drummond *et al.*, 1997), and these are briefly described in Table 1. Whilst several cost-of-illness studies of epilepsy have recently been presented (Cockerell *et al.*, 1994; Beran and Banks, 1995; Cockerell *et al.*, 1995; Gessner *et al.*, 1995; van Hout *et al.*, 1997; Jacoby *et al.*, 1998), other types of economic appraisal of epilepsy or epilepsy treatment are rare. Types of economic evaluation in epilepsy have included a cost-effectiveness comparison of adjunctive antiepileptic drugs (O'Neill *et al.*, 1995); a cost-minimization study of four antiepileptic drugs used in monotherapy for newly diagnosed patients with epilepsy (Heaney *et al.*, 1995); a cost-minimization analysis comparing carbamazepine and lamotrigine (Shakespeare and Simeon, 1998); a cost-effectiveness model of adjunctive lamotrigine (Markowitz *et al.*, 1998) and a life-time cost–utility analysis of adjunctive lamotrigine therapy in patients with refractory seizures (Messori *et al.*, 1998).

Table 1. Types of economic evaluation.

Evaluation type	Use
Cost-of-illness studies (COI)	To itemize, value and sum the costs of a particular problem with the aim of giving an idea of its economic burden
Cost-minimization analysis (CMA)	If the interventions have the same consequences, the economic analysis can concentrate on inputs only. This analysis is concerned with the identification of the intervention with the lowest possible costs.
Cost-effectiveness analysis (CEA)	If the outcome of interest is the same in two programmes, but there is different success in achieving the outcome.
Cost-benefit analysis (CBA)	If neither the consequences not the outcomes of two programmes are the same. CBA aims to compare all social costs and consequences across different interventions or against a 'do nothing' option.
Cost–utility analysis (CUA)	This analysis is preferred by analysts who have reservations about valuing benefits in dollar terms. Utility refers to the preferences individuals or society may have for any particular set of health outcomes. This approach incorporates *quality of life* adjustments to treatment outcomes.

In the cost–utility study (Messori *et al.*, 1998), although some of the data, the QOL values, were obtained prospectively by interviewing a group of patients, the main analysis was based on estimates taken from the published literature.

All of these studies used some form of pharmacoeconomic decision-analytic model based on a number of assumptions and estimates using data from various sources, such as clinical trial data, expert clinical opinion and published literature.

Decision-analytic models have been developed because data on the pharmacoeconomic aspects of medical treatment in general, and epilepsy in particular, are extremely scant. Whilst health economists' methods include extensive use of models, it is argued that the conclusions of such studies are unsatisfactory, and a move away from such modelling in health care has been predicted (Drummond, 1996).

Given the limitations of decision-analytic, pharmacoeconomic models, a prospective, follow-up study was conducted to compare the outcome and costs of patients who were about to start one of a number of the newer adjunctive antiepileptic drugs. The aim was to collect data on outcome and costs and to compare these to data generated by a pharmacoeconomic model. Another aim was to collect QOL data using two methods: (1) an individualized technique and (2) an instrument developed within the psychometric and econometric traditions. A cost-effective analysis of two antiepileptic drugs, lamotrigine and topiramate, was previously reported (Selai *et al.*, 1999). Here, a cost-effectiveness analysis is presented of four adjunctive antiepileptic drugs: clobazam, lamotrigine, gabapentin and vigabatrin.

MATERIAL AND METHODS

Patients about to start on one of the four adjunctive antiepileptic drugs (clobazam, lamotrigine, vigabatrin and gabapentin) were approached after their medical consultation in the outpatient clinic, and the study was explained to them. Patients who were willing to take part were offered the choice of a telephone interview at home (for convenience) as an alternative to a face-to-face interview at the hospital, and most patients chose this option. The timing of the interviews was: (1) baseline; (2) 3 months from baseline; and (3) 6 months from baseline.

Costings incorporated in the study

Resource uses and their costs have traditionally been divided into 'direct costs' and 'indirect costs' or 'productivity costs' in the literature (Luce *et al.*, 1996). Direct costs include the value of all goods, services and other resources that are consumed in the provision of an intervention or in dealing with the side effects and other sequelae. Direct costs encompass all types of resource use, including the consumption of professional, family, volunteer, or patient time. Direct healthcare costs include the costs of tests, drugs, supplies, health-care personnel and medical facilities. Direct non-healthcare costs include transportation costs to and from the clinic and child care fees. The two types of costs that comprise indirect costs or productivity costs are (1) the costs associated with lost or impaired ability to work or to engage in leisure activities due to illness and (2) lost economic productivity due to death.

This study restricted the analysis to the direct costs of medication and the costs of direct sequelae such as side effects or adverse events that required medical attention and therefore incurred a cost. The costs of medical personnel incurred during the epilepsy outpatient clinic visits, the opportunity costs of the patient taking time off work and the transportation costs from home to the clinic were not calculated.

MAIN OUTCOME MEASURES

The National Hospital Seizure Severity Scale (O'Donoghue et al., 1996)

This was used to assess seizure frequency and seizure severity. This scale is administered by a health professional during an interview with both the patient and a witness to the seizures. It contains seven seizure-related factors and generates a score from 1 to 27.

Drug-related sequelae

Side effects, adverse events and reason for stopping medication were also recorded.

Quality of life

QOL was measured by the Quality of Life Assessment Schedule (QOLAS) (Kendrick and Trimble, 1994) and the EuroQol instrument (EuroQol Group, 1990; Brooks, 1996). The QOLAS results were previously reported by Selai and Trimble (1998); the EuroQol EQ-5D data are reported by Selai and colleagues (unpublished results).

QOLAS

Quality of Life Assessment Schedule (QOLAS) is an individualized QOL assessment technique tailored to each individual patient, and is a revised version of the QoLASCA, a method originally based on RGT (McGuire, 1991; Kendrick and Trimble, 1994; Kendrick, 1997). The full QoLASCA technique was somewhat burdensome and the revised method (QOLAS) has been considerably streamlined. Two main aspects of the original theoretical work have been maintained: (1) the original emphasis (in order to assess therapeutic outcome) on a careful and comprehensive interview, recording items of importance to the patient in the patient's own words; (2) the idea that QOL is a function of the conceptual distance between 'how I am now' and 'how I would like to be' – the gap between actuality and expectation. This is known in the medical literature as 'Calman's gap' because Calman suggested that a key aim of medical care should be to narrow the gap between a patient's hopes and expectations and what actually happens (Calman, 1984).

QOLAS interview

The QOLAS interview used in this study is as follows:
1. Introduction and rapport-building.
2. The respondent is invited to recount what is important for his/her QOL and ways in which his/her current health condition is affecting QOL. Key constructs are extracted from this narrative. Prompting is sometimes required.
3. In total, 10 'constructs' are elicited, two for each of the following domains of QOL: physical, psychological, social, daily activities and cognitive functioning (or well-being).
4. The patient is asked to rate how much of a problem each of these is now on a 0–5 scale, where 0 = no problem; 1 = very slight problem; 2 = mild problem; 3 = moderate problem; 4 = big problem; and 5 = it could not be worse.
5. The patient is asked to rate how much of a problem they would like each of these to be on the same 0–5 scale.
6. At follow-up interview, the respondent's individual constructs are read out to them and they are invited to re-rate each on the 0–5 scale for how much of a problem there is with each *now*.

QOLAS scoring

1. For each construct, the *like* score is subtracted from the *now* score, giving a score for the distance between expectation and reality.
2. The scores, calculated in (1) directly above, for the two constructs per domain are summed to give a domain score out of 10. The total for each of the five domains is summed to give an overall QOLAS score out of 50.

Patient satisfaction

Patient satisfaction was operationally defined. Patients were 'satisfied' if they fulfilled all of the following criteria: (1) still on drug at $t = 3$; (2) experiencing no side effects; (3) had no adverse events; and (4) had a greater than 50% reduction in seizures.

Costs

Patients were asked at follow-up interviews for dates of stopping medication. The costs for the three drugs included in the pharmacoeconomic paper (O'Neill *et al.*, 1995) were taken from that paper. The costs for gabapentin, which were not calculated in that paper, were taken from *MIMS* 1995 so that these costs corresponded with the 1995 costs. Costs relating to adverse events were obtained from the OHE *Compendium of Health Statistics* (OHE, 1989), from health authority sources and from other public bodies as appropriate. Costs were calculated on an 'intention to treat' basis (Pocock, 1983) and so, for the group of patients who were lost to follow-up, data concerning their continuation (or otherwise) with medication were taken from the patients' notes. The costs of medication for these patients were thus included, but data on side effects and adverse events were not included because interviews had not been completed and these data were not systemically recorded in the patients' notes.

Costs of 'adverse events'

In the operational definition of 'satisfaction', all epilepsy-related adverse events were included because these had an impact on compliance and QOL. For the cost-effectiveness comparison, however, only those events were included where medical advice was sought and a cost was therefore incurred. An example of such an event is the development of a skin rash that resulted in extra GP and/or clinic visits.

Cost-effectiveness comparison

In order to compare the cost-effectiveness of the different drugs, the cost-effectiveness ratio published in the pharmacoeconomic paper was used. The formula is as follows:

CER = cost per successfully treated patient

$$= \frac{\text{cost per patient per treatment}}{\text{\% successfully treated patients}}$$

RESULTS: PART 1 – DESCRIPTIVE

A total of 97 patients were recruited into the study. Of these, 78 attended for both follow-up interviews and 19 failed to attend follow-up. Those lost to follow up were incorporated and an 'intention to treat analysis' was performed. The full outcome of those patients who started on the four drugs and who completed all three interviews ($n = 78$) is reported; the 19 patients who were lost to follow-up are incorporated into the cost-effectiveness analysis.

Of the 78 patients, 15 started on vigabatrin (of which 10 were male), 20 on clobazam (8 male), 26 on lamotrigine (14 male) and 17 on gabapentin (8 male).

Of the 19 patients lost to follow-up, three had started on vigabatrin, four on clobazam, six on gabapentin and six on lamotrigine.

Seizures at baseline

Most of the patients had either non-convulsive seizures or both convulsions and other seizure types. Of the 78 patients, 31 (40%) patients were experiencing convulsive seizures. Only three patients (all on vigabatrin) were experiencing convulsions exclusively. The number experiencing convulsions for each drug was six on vigabatrin, seven on clobazam, 13 on lamotrigine and five on gabapentin.

First follow-up interview ($t = 2$)

At the 3-month follow-up, 13 patients were still on vigabatrin (87%), 14 were still on clobazam (70%), 21 were still on lamotrigine (81%) and 14 remained on gabapentin (82%).

Status at $t = 3$ interview

Table 2 shows individual data for the 78 patients at the 6-month follow-up. The side effects reported by the patients are shown in Appendix 1.

Table 2. Individual data for patients at the 6-month follow-up.

Status at 6 months	Vigabatrin	Clobazam	Lamotrigine	Gabapentin	Total
Still on drug	10/15	08/20	16/26	10/17	44/78
Experiencing side effects[a]	7/15	3/20	10/26	6/17	26/78
Experienced serious adverse events[b]	1/15	4/20	1/26	5/17	11/78
50% or more reduction in seizures	8/15	6/20	10/26	7/17	31/78
No. patients 'satisfied'[c]	4/15	4/20	3/26	2/17	13/78
Did not attend follow-up interview	3	4	6	6	19

[a]Side effects as reported by patients and attributed by them to the add-on therapy;
[b]Serious adverse events are epilepsy-related events requiring urgent medical intervention;
[c]Operational criteria for 'satisfied' were: (1) still on drug at $t = 3$; (2) experiencing no side effects; (3) had no adverse events; and (4) had a greater than 50% reduction in seizures.

Table 3. Costs (£) for the 6-month period of starting patients on each of the four drugs.

	Total therapy (n = 78)	(n = 20)	Adverse events (n = 78)	Total cost (£)	Cost/ patient
Vigabatrin (n = 18)	4424	446	1178	6048	336
Clobazam (n = 24)	1969	91	3099	5159	215
Lamotrigine (n = 32)	10 111	1377	7303	18 791	587
Gabapentin (n = 23)	4348	928	10 181	15 457	672

RESULTS: PART 2 – COSTINGS (DRUGS AND INDIRECT COSTS)

The costs of the drugs for the 6-month period are shown in Table 3. The total costs divided by the number of patients 'satisfied' are shown in Table 4. Table 5 shows the cost-effectiveness of these drugs compared with data obtained from the published pharmacoeconomic model. Two sets of costs were calculated: (1) the costs of drug therapy taken from both the previous pharmacoeconomic paper and *MIMS* and (2) the indirect medical costs relating to adverse events, costs for which were obtained from various health authorities and public sources.

Table 4. Costs of starting patients on each drug, divided by number of patients 'satisfied' at the end of the 6-month follow-up period.

Drug	No. satisfied	% Satisfied	Total cost/no. of 'satisfied' patients
Vigabatrin (n = 18)	4	22	1512
Clobazam (n = 24)	4	17	1290
Lamotrigine (n = 32)	3	9	6264
Gabapentin (n = 23)	2	9	7729

Table 5. Cost-effectiveness comparison of each of the four drugs.

	6/12	12/12	% Satisfied	Audit	Pharmacoeconomic model
Vigabatrin	336 × 2 = 672/		22 =	31	14.47
Clobazam	215 × 2 = 430/		17 =	25	10.34
Lamotrigine	587 × 2 = 1174/		9 =	130	14.79
Gabapentin	672 × 2 = 1344/		9 =	149	–

RESULTS: PART 3 – QOLAS DATA

Figure 1 shows the total QOLAS scores at baseline and at the 6-month follow-up for two subgroups of patients. The group deemed 'satisfied'

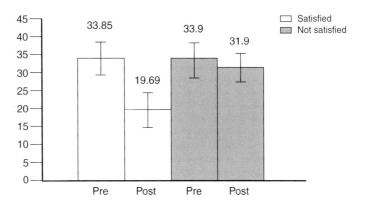

Figure 1. Total Quality of Life Assessment Schedule scores for the two groups: 'satisfied' (white bars) ($n = 13$) and 'unsatisfied' (shaded bars) ($n = 10$) at baseline and at 6 month follow-up. The error bars show 95% confidence intervals. The pre- and post-scores for the two groups were compared using paired t-tests. The scores for the satisfied group were statistically significantly different, $t = 6.78$, $p > 0.0001$.
(Reproduced, with permission, from Selai and Trimble, 1998.)

according to the operational definition ($n = 13$) showed a significant improvement in QOL; two-tailed paired t-tests, $t = 6.78$, $p < 0.0001$. The second group in Figure 1, labelled 'not satisfied', is a subset who did not achieve a > 50% reduction in seizures and were experiencing side effects, and had experienced an adverse event at $t = 0.91$, $p < 0.384$.

DISCUSSION

In this study an audit was carried out of patients treated with one of four adjunctive anticonvulsant drugs. Of the patients who were still on the 'new' drug at the 6-month follow-up, only 17% reported being satisfied (according to the operational definition), i.e. had > 50% seizure reduction and were experiencing neither side effects nor adverse events. Although many studies identify patients who have achieved a reduction in seizure frequency, few emphasize QOL measures of patient satisfaction. The fact that only 17% of patients were satisfied helps to explain why Walker and colleagues found that 86% of patients in long-term follow-up had stopped taking the drugs (Walker *et al.*, 1996).

It could be argued that our definition of 'satisfied' is too harsh. The most controversial aspect would be the inclusion of side effects as opposed to more significant adverse events in this measure. However, the clinical reality is that patients are concerned about the side effects, want to discuss them with the researcher, and it is generally accepted that they are a central feature of QOL, or satisfaction with treatment, for patients taking these drugs (Cramer, 1994). The QOL scores, as assessed by QOLAS, showed that only those patients 'satisfied' had significantly improved QOL scores at the 6-months follow-up. These data emphasize that future studies of antiepilepsy drugs need to tease out the complicated effects of seizure relief, side effects and adverse events upon patient-perceived QOL, and not just measure the 50% or greater reduction seizures as is usually the case in the current literature.

In appraising this study, a number of methodological points need to be considered. First, this is a naturalistic study and not a clinical trial. Whilst clinical trials yield important data, they tend to use highly selected patients, rarely examine issues of QOL, and the data may simply not be generalizable to the clinical setting.

Secondly, this study considers the cost-effectiveness of *starting* patients on each of the four drugs. The cost-effectiveness ratio alters according to the choice of outcome criteria: a different picture is obtained of the relationships between the drugs depending upon whether only the cost of therapy is considered or whether patient satisfaction is taken into account.

Thirdly, an attempt has been made to at least partially replicate a pharmacoeconomic study, although that considered a period of 1 year. The present study was over 6 months, but the data were adjusted for comparison with the published data for 1-year period. This may have influenced the cost-effectiveness ratios. However, when the cost-effectiveness ratios between the drugs in this study and that based only on a model are compared, there are clearly substantial differences and it is unlikely that adjusting the data wholly accounts for the observed differences. There are a number of reasons for these differences, not least being that the present model, and, as far as the authors are aware, most published models, fail to incorporate patient 'satisfaction' in the same way. This raises doubts about the value of using existing models to evaluate different therapies.

Sensitivity analysis

Whilst guidelines for papers on economic topics recommend the inclusion of a sensitivity analysis (Drummond *et al.*, 1997), where certain chosen variables are varied (Briggs *et al.*, 1994), such an analysis has not been undertaken here because the current study has looked at the clinical reality rather than an estimate of costs. In both this study and a previous cost-effectiveness paper (Selai *et al.*, 1999), methodological issues surrounding the choice of what epilepsy-related costs to include are discussed.

Finally, it should be pointed out that there are no guidelines regarding what 'events' should be included in the costing, although a recent paper makes some recommendations concerning which costs to include in epilepsy cost-of-illness studies (Begley *et al.*, 1999). There are no clear criteria for distinguishing between a cost incurred as a direct result of being on a particular drug and a cost which is, arguably, a more general cost of having epilepsy. This study has included epilepsy-related events such as magnetic resonance image scans, GP visits and hospital admissions, but has excluded certain other events, an example being the cost of radiotherapy for a brain tumour. Decisions concerning the costing of the events can be criticized, but there are no gold standards by which inclusions and exclusions can be established and the suggestion has been made that guidelines need to be drawn up (Spilker, 1996).

The discrepancy between the clinical audit and the published data highlights the need for caution in deriving data from pharmacoeconomic models. In particular, cost-effectiveness studies of antiepileptic drugs need to take account of adverse events, which often have important resource implications.

CONCLUSIONS

This audit conducted at a tertiary referral centre suggests that only a minority of patients with intractable epilepsy going on to the newer anticonvulsants derive substantial treatment benefit from these drugs when given as an add-on therapy. The higher costs of the newer agents plus the high costs relating to adverse events have important implications for the continued debate concerning the most effective use of scarce health resources.

ACKNOWLEDGEMENTS

For assistance with recruitment of patients we gratefully acknowledge: Professor S. Shorvon, Professor J. Duncan, Professor J.W.A. Sander, Professor D. Fish and Dr S. Smith. Thanks also to Dr M. O'Donoghue who provided training in the use of the National Hospital Seizure Severity Scale.

Appendix 1. Side effects reported by patients at t = 2 and/or t = 3 (patients may experience more than one side effect).

Side effects	Vigabatrin	Clobazam	Lamotrigine	Gabapentin
Psychological/behavioural change	–	8	5	2
Drowsiness	4	5	2	4
Cognitive	4	2	6	2
Skin rash	–	–	3	–
Light headed/dizziness	1	2	1	3
Nausea/vomiting	–	–	–	2
Headache	1	1	3	1
Weight gain	2	1	2	1
Weight loss	–	–	1	–
Diplopia/other visual	–	1	4	4
Tremor	–	–	2	–
Stagger/balance/ataxia	1	2	–	1
Limb pain/swelling	2	–	–	1
Gums bleeding (worse)	1	–	–	–
Sense of taste lost	–	1	–	–
Unbearable itching	–	1	–	–
Bruising	–	1	1	–
Runny nose	–	–	1	–
Urinary incontinence	–	–	2	–
Stiffness	–	–	1	–
Sexual performance	–	–	–	1
Hot flushes	–	–	–	1
Menstrual problems	–	–	–	1

REFERENCES

Begley, C.E., Annegers, J.F., Lairson, D.R. and Reynolds, T.F. (1999). Methodological issues in estimating the cost of epilepsy. *Epilepsy Res* **33**, 39–55.

Beran, R.G. and Banks, G.K. (1995). Indirect costs of epilepsy in Australia. In: Beran, R.G. and Pachlatko, C.P. (Eds), *Cost of Epilepsy: Proceedings of the 20th International Epilepsy Congress.* Ciba-Geigy Verlag, Wehr/Baden, pp. 49–54.

Brazier, J. and Deverill, M. (1999). A checklist for judging preference-based measures of health related quality of life: learning from psychometrics. *Health Econ* **8**, 41–51.

Briggs, A., Sculpher, M. and Buxton, M. (1994). Uncertainty in the economic evaluation of health care technologies: the role of sensitivity analysis. *Health Econ* **3**, 95–104.

Brooks, R. (1996). EuroQol: The current state of play. *Health Pol* **37**, 53–72.

Calman, K.C. (1984). Quality of life in cancer patients – a hypothesis. *J Med Ethics* **10**, 124–127.

Cockerell, O.C., Hart, Y.M., Sander, J.W.A.S. and Shorvon, S.D. (1994). The cost of epilepsy in the United Kingdom: an estimation based on the results of two population-based studies. *Epilepsy Res* **18**, 249–260.

Cockerell, O.C., Hart, Y.M., Sander, J.W.A.S. and Shorvon, S.D. (1995). The cost of epilepsy in the U.K. In: Beran, R.G. and Pachlatko, C.P. (Eds), *Cost of Epilepsy: Proceedings of the 20th International Epilepsy Congress.* Ciba-Geigy Verlag, Wehr/Baden, pp. 27–37.

Cramer, J. (1994). Quality of life and compliance. In: Trimble, M.R. and Dodson, W.E. (Eds), *Epilepsy and the Quality of Life*. Raven Press, New York, pp. 49–63.

Cramer, J. (1996). Quality of life assessment for people with epilepsy. In: Spilker, B. (Ed.), *Quality of Life and Pharmacoeconomics in Clinical Trials, 2nd edn.* Lippincott-Raven, Philadelphia, pp. 909–918.

Drummond, M.F. (1996). The future of pharmacoeconomics. In: Spilker, B. (Ed.), *Quality of Life and Pharmacoeconomics in Clinical Trials, 2nd edn.* Lippincott-Raven, Philadelphia, pp. 1225–1228.

Drummond, M.F., O'Brien, B., Stoddart, G.L. and Torrance, G.W. (1997). *Methods for the Economic Evaluation of Health Care Programmes (2nd edn).* Oxford University Press, Oxford.

EuroQol Group (1990). EuroQol – a new facility for the measurement of health-related quality of life. *Health Pol* **16**, 199–208.

Fransella, F. and Bannister, D. (1977). *A Manual for Repertory Grid Technique*. Academic Press, Harcourt Brace Jovanovich, London.

Fraser, S.C.A., Ramirez, A.J., Ebbs, S.R. *et al.* (1993). A Daily Diary Card for Quality of Life Measurement in Advanced Breast Cancer Trials. *Br J Cancer* **67**, 341–346.

Geddes, D.M., Dones, L., Hill, E. *et al.* (1990). Quality of life during chemotherapy for small cell lung cancer: assessment and use of a daily diary card in a randomised trial. *Eur J Cancer* **26**, 484–492.

Gessner, U., Sagmeister, M. and Horisberger, B. (1995). The economic impact of epilepsy in Switzerland. In: Beran, R.G. and Pachlatko, C.P. (Eds), *Cost of Epilepsy: Proceedings of the 20th International Epilepsy Congress*. Ciba-Geigy Verlag, Wehr/Baden, pp. 67–74.

Gill, T.M. (1995). Quality of Life Assessment: values and pitfalls. *J R Soc Med* **88**, 680–682.

Gill, T.M. and Feinstein, A.R. (1994). A critical appraisal of the quality of life measurements. *JAMA* **272**, 619–626.

Gold, M.R., Siegel, J.E., Russell, L.B. and Weinstein, M.C. (Eds) (1996). *Cost-effectiveness in Health and Medicine*. Oxford University Press, Oxford.

Guyatt, G.H., Berman, L.B., Townsend, M., Pugsley, S.O. and Chambers, L.W. (1987a). A measure of quality of life for clinical trials in chronic lung disease. *Thorax* **42**, 773–778.

Guyatt, G.H., Townsend, M., Pugsley, S.O. *et al.* (1987b). Bronchodilators in chronic air-flow limitation. *Am Rev Respir Dis* **135**, 1069–1074.

Heaney, D.C., Shorvon, S.D. and Sander, J.W. (1995). An economic appraisal of carbamazepine, lamotrigine, phenytoin and valporate as initial treatment in adults with newly diagnosed epilepsy. *Epilepsia* **39** (suppl 3), S19–S25.

Hedrick, S.C., Taeuber, R.C. and Erickson, P. (1996). On learning and understanding quality of life: a guide to information sources. In: Spilker, B. (Ed.), *Quality of Life and Pharmacoeconomics in Clinical Trials, 2nd edn.* Lippincott-Raven, Philadelphia, pp. 59–64.

Jacoby, A., Buck, D., Baker, G., McNamee, P., Graham-Jones, S. and Chadwick, D. (1998). Uptake and costs for epilepsy: findings from a UK regional study. *Epilepsia* **39**, 776–786.

Jefferson, T., Demicheli, V. and Mugford, M. (1996). *Elementary Economic Evaluation in Health Care*. BMJ Publishing Group, London.

Juniper, E.F., Guyatt, G.H. and Jaeschke, R. (1996). How to develop and validate a new health-related quality of life instrument. In: Spilker, B. (Ed.), *Quality of Life and Pharmacoeconomics in Clinical Trials, 2nd edn.* Lippincott-Raven, Philadelphia, pp. 49–56.

Kendrick, A. (1997). Quality of life. In: Cull, C. and Goldstein, L.H. (Eds), *The Clinical Psychologist's Handbook of Epilepsy*. Routledge, London and New York, pp. 130–148.

Kendrick, A.M. and Trimble, M.R. (1994). Repertory grid in the assessment of quality of life in patients with epilepsy: The Quality of Life Assessment Schedule. In: Trimble, M.R. and Dodson, W.E. (Eds), *Epilepsy and the Quality of Life*. Raven Press, New York, pp. 151–163.

Luce, B.R., Manning, W.G., Siegel, J.E. and Lipscomb, J. (1996). Estimating the costs in cost-effectiveness analysis. In: Gold, M.R., Siegel, J.E., Russell, L.B. and Weinstein, M.C. (Eds), *Cost-effectiveness in Health and Medicine*. Oxford University Press, Oxford, pp. 176–213.

Markowitz, M.A., Mauskopf, J.A. and Halpern, M.T. (1998). Cost-effectiveness model of adjunctive lamotrigine for the treatment of epilepsy. *Neurology* **51**, 1026–1033.

Mays, N. and Pope, C. (1996). Rigour and qualitative research. In: Mays, N. and Pope, C. (Eds), *Qualitative Research in Health Care*. BMJ Publishing Group, London, pp. 10–19.

McDonnell, G.V. and Morrow, J.I. (1996). An audit of the new antiepileptic drugs in clinical neurological practice. *Seizure* **5**, 127–130.

McDowell, I. and Newell, C. (1987). *Measuring Health: A Guide to Rating Scales and Questionnaires*. Oxford University Press, Oxford, New York.

McGuire, A.M. (1991). Quality of life in women with epilepsy. In: Trimble, M.R. (Ed.), *Women and Epilepsy*. John Wiley, Chichester, pp. 13–30.

Messori, A., Trippoli, S., Becagli, P., Cincotta, M., Labbate, M.G. and Zaccara, G. (1998). Adjunctive lamotrigine therapy in patients with refractory seizures: a lifetime cost-utility analysis. *J Clin Pharmacol* **53**, 421–427.

O'Boyle, C.A., McGee, H.M., Hickey, A. *et al.* (1993). *The Schedule for the Evaluation of Individual Quality of Life (SEIQoL)*. Administration manual. Department of Psychology, Royal College of Surgeons in Ireland, Dublin.

O'Donoghue, M.F., Duncan, J.S. and Sander, J.W.A.S. (1996). The National Hospital Seizure Severity Scale: a further development of the Chalfont Seizure Severity Scale. *Epilepsia* **37**, 563–571.

Office of Health Economics (1989). *Compendium of Health Statistics* (7th edn). Office of Health Economics, London.

O'Neill, B.A., Trimble, M.R. and Bloom, D.S. (1995). Adjunctive therapy in epilepsy: a cost-effectiveness comparison of alternative treatment options. *Seizure* **4**, 37–44.

Pocock, S.J. (1983). *Clinical Trials: A Practical Approach*. John Wiley, Chichester.

Ruta, D.A., Garratt, A.M., Leng, M., Russel, I.T. and MacDonald, L.M. (1994). A new approach to the measurement of quality of life: the patient-generated index (PGI). *Med Care* **32**, 1109–1126.

Selai, C.E. and Trimble, M.R. (1998). Adjunctive therapy in epilepsy with new antiepileptic drugs: is it of any value. *Seizure* **7**, 417–418.

Selai, C.E., Smith, K. and Trimble, M.R. (1999). Adjunctive therapy in epilepsy: a cost-effectiveness comparison of two AEDs. *Seizure* **8**, 8–13.

Selai, C.E., Trimble, M.R., Rossor, M. and Harvey, R. (2000). The feasibility and validity of the Quality of Life Assessment Schedule (QOLAS) in patients with dementia. *J Neuropsychol Rehab* in press.

Shakespeare, A. and Simeon, G. (1998). Economic analysis of epilepsy treatment: a cost minimisation analysis comparing carbamazepine and lamotrigine in the UK. *Seizure* **7**, 119–125.

Shorvon, S. (1997). Antiepileptic drug monotherapy versus polytherapy: economic aspects. *Epilepsia* **38** (suppl 5), S17–S20.

Spilker, B. (1996). Developing guidelines for pharmacoeconomic trials. In: Spilker, B. (Ed.), *Quality of Life and Pharmacoeconomics in Clinical Trials*, 2nd edn. Lippincott-Raven, Philadelphia, pp. 1123–1130.

Trimble, M.R. and Dodson, W.E. (Eds) (1994). *Epilepsy and the Quality of Life.* Raven Press, New York.

Tugwell, P., Bombardier, C., Buchanan, W.W. *et al.* (1990). Methotrexate in rheumatoid arthritis: impact on quality of life assessed by traditional standard item and individualized patient preference health status questionnaires. *Arch Intern Med* **150**, 59–82.

van Hout, B., Gagnon, D., Souetre, E. *et al.* (1997). Relationship between seizure frequency and costs and quality of life of outpatients with partial epilepsy in France, Germany, and the United Kingdom. *Epilepsia* **38**, 1221–1226.

Vickrey, B.G. (1995). Advances in the measurement of health-related quality of life in epilepsy. *J Qual Life Res* **8**, 83–85.

Walker, M.C., Li, L.M. and Sander, J.W.A.S. (1996). Long-term use of lamotrigine and vigabatrin in severe refractory epilepsy: audit of outcome. *BMJ* **313**, 1184–1185.

13

The Benzodiazepine Addiction Story

CHRISTER ALLGULANDER

*Karolinska Institutet, Department of Clinical Neuroscience and Family Medicine,
Division of Psychiatry, Huddinge University Hospital, Huddinge, Sweden*

INTRODUCTION

The purpose of this chapter is to give a perspective on the literature regarding the propensity of benzodiazepines to be misused.

The benzodiazepine class of drugs stems from the heptoxdiazines which where discovered in 1891. The first medication to be approved by the Food and Drug Administration in 1960 was chlordiazepoxide (Librium) followed by diazepam (Valium) in 1963 and then oxazepam in 1965. By 1990, there were 34 benzodiazepines in clinical use.

The most common indication for benzodiazepines is insomnia, particularly in the elderly, when caused by anxiety/depression, brain lesional syndromes, painful rheumatic conditions, congestive heart failure or bereavement (Hollister *et al.*, 1993; Bell and Nutt, 1995). Benzodiazepines are also used to attenuate withdrawal symptoms from alcohol, including delirium tremens. They are effective as adjuvants to neuroleptics in coping with agitation in acute mania or psychosis in inpatient psychiatric units. In neurological patients, they are used to terminate grand mal seizures and acute muscular tension such as torticollis. They are also indicated for maintenance therapy in seizure disorders, and in spasticity.

FROM WINE TO MINOR TRANQUILLIZERS

Mankind has always used alcohol for its anxiolytic and hypnotic properties. Wine and opium, or natural remedies such as castor, camphor and valeriana were used by the ancient Greeks, Egyptians, Arabs and Romans. The use of warm oil on shaven heads to fume out vapours in the insane was still condoned in the late 1800s. Paracelsus (1493–1541) advocated iron filings to hysteric patients, a treatment still recommended in the USA in 1890. With the isolating of morphine in 1816 and the invention of the hypodermic needle in 1853, opiate therapy became a panacea, particularly in mentally disordered patients. Bromide was discovered in sea water in 1826, and in 1872 it was reported to relieve insomnia and excitement.

A turning point was the introduction in 1903 of the first barbituric acid for sedation and sleep. Bromide and a number of barbituric derivatives became the backbone of such therapy, with 20 daily doses per 1000 inhabitants in Sweden in 1947 (Allgulander, 1986). The Swedish pharmacopea in 1953 reported seven opioid concoctions, 17 barbituric formulations, two with bromide, three with valeriana and one with chloral hydrate. In the mid-1950s, subsequent to the breakthrough of chlorpromazine treatment in psychotic patients, a number of new sedative/hypnotics were introduced (methaqualone, meprobamate, ethinamate, ethchlorvynol, clomethiazole, glutethimide, methyprylone, propiomazine, promethazine).

MISUSE OF SEDATIVE–HYPNOTICS

Case reports of misuse of sedative-hypnotics appeared in the late 1800s and following the introduction of most of the compounds in 1950s. Systematic clinical studies of such patients appeared first in Paris (Le Guillant, 1930), and Leipzig (Pohlisch and Panse, 1934). Clinicians found shared psychiatric denominators among sedative–hypnotic misusers prior to the introduction of the benzodiazepines; in Norway (Retterstöl and Sund, 1964), Sweden (Allgulander *et al.*, 1987), Switzerland (Wissler, 1969), Australia (Whitlock, 1970), Minnesota (Swanson *et al.*, 1973) and Denmark (Nimb, 1975).

Most striking about these patients were long histories of severe psychiatric symptoms, and maladaptive personality traits which preceded the prescribing of a range of psychoactive medications with differing pharmacodynamic properties. Ljungberg (1957) identified hysteria as a risk diagnosis. As a group, patients addicted or dependent on sedative–hypnotics had in common gross, often antisocial, psychopathology prior to treatment, conducive to a need for voluntary or involuntary inpatient detoxification due to physical and mental withdrawal symptoms from overdosing medications. These symptoms included seizures and delirium. The patients often resumed a self-destructive lifestyle with a high tendency to relapse and to commit suicide. Many denied having exceeded prescribed doses, even after hospital admission for pathognomonic withdrawal symptoms.

High doses were usually obtained by seeing several practitioners concomitantly, exploiting the confidentiality of physician treatment and pharmacy handling, and violating the trust of the physicians – one not knowing what the other was doing. Other means of obtaining high doses were stealing from hospital supplies; forging and altering of prescriptions; smuggling in used, labelled pill bottles; and prescribing by proxy, i.e. colluding with a spouse or friend posing as a patient with simulated symptoms. Similar patterns of acquisition have been noted among subjects abusing benzodiazepines in a recent report from the Psychopharmacology Committee of the Royal College of Psychiatrists (1997).

The risk of verified suicide was particularly high among doctors, nurses and pharmacists who had become addicted to prescription drugs prior to the benzodiazepines (Nimb, 1975; Allgulander *et al.*, 1987). The potentially lethal toxicity of the barbiturates and other such medications was a great concern to physicians at the time.

THE BENZODIAZEPINE REVOLUTION

The heralding of meprobamate in 1955 as a non-toxic alternative to the barbiturates turned out to be wrong. Thus, chlordiazepoxide, diazepam, nitrazepam and oxazepam were received with caution in the mid-1960s. But the superior risk/benefit ratio over those of available sedative–hypnotics was quickly noted. The benzodiazepines turned out to be a major improvement in the treatment of anxiety and sleep disorders. The legislation that emerged in 1960–62 following the thalidomide disaster provided a firm basis for assessing the efficacy and safety of this new treatment. Controlled studies of benzodiazepines were, however, done with patients suffering from psychoneurosis, an ambiguous psychodynamic term.

Sweden saw the number of doses of the total sedative–hypnotic–anxiolytic class of medications rising substantially with the marketing of diazepam, nitrazepam and oxazepam, peaking in 1972 at 66 daily doses per 1000 inhabitants. Two-thirds of the benzodiazepine doses were to treat patients with insomnia.

Physicians in the 1960s ventured to treat nervous patients more liberally in the absence of formal diagnoses. Psychiatric diagnosing was becoming politically incorrect with the activist trend to declare mental illness a myth used for social repression. It was only in 1980 with DSM-III that psychoneurosis, introduced in 1769 by the neurologist William Cullen, began its exodus from the treatment studies and the pharmacopeas to be replaced with the current nosology for anxiety syndromes resting on operationalized criteria.

EARLY WARNING

The risk of suicide with benzodiazepines was negligible compared with that of the barbiturates. But the number of self-poisonings with prescribed medications rose in the late 1960s in Sweden, causing concern over too liberal prescribing of benzodiazepines. In 1971, Sweden legally classified the benzo-diazepines as narcotics. This received media attention, fuelling attacks on psychoactive medications in general; and the benzodiazepines in particular. The populistic groups against street drugs welcomed this addition, joining force with some government authorities and advocates of psychodynamic psychotherapy.

The benzodiazepines vastly expanded the exposure among the public in Europe to psychoactive medications. This caused mixed feelings in the professional community. Contemporary thought-leaders were influenced by the 'Zeitgeist'. Ideström (1969) wrote: 'The question is whether contaminat-ing the "internal environment" with anxiolytics and hypnotics can be compared with contaminating the external environment with mercury and insecticides'. Lader (1978) entitled a paper 'The benzodiazepines – the opium of the masses?'. The Danish psychoanalyst Vanggaard (1988) exclaimed that 'Daytime benzodiazepines, in my opinion, are the Devil's work'. Kräupl Taylor (1989) followed this lead with a paper on 'The damnation of benzo-diazepines'.

IDEOLOGICAL VIGILANCE CONTRA MOLECULAR FINDINGS

The libertarian psychiatrist/anti-psychiatrist Thomas Szasz (1974), honorary member of the scientology business unit Citizens Commission for Human Rights, opined that: 'Trying to understand drug addiction by studying drugs makes as much sense as trying to understand holy water by studying water'.

Oddly, this sarcasm is relevant when it comes to understanding the driving forces of benzodiazepine misuse. While ignoring the characteristics of patients misusing prescription drugs, debaters focused on the pharmaco-dynamic properties. There is now a growing consensus that certain individ-uals are at high risk of abusing benzodiazepines and other compounds (World Health Organization, 1996; Royal College of Psychiatrists, 1997).

Experts reviewing human and animal studies of the pharmacology of benzodiazepines did not find conclusive evidence that they are addictive. Their findings can be divided into three domains: reinforcement, physical dependence, and tolerance.

Reinforcement

Two extensive reviews of the pharmacology of benzodiazepines were done by Woods and colleagues (1987, 1992). They concluded that there was 'a striking finding of absence of reinforcing effect in normal subject groups representing the populations for which benzodiazepines are most frequently prescribed'. A similar conclusion was drawn by clinical and pharmacological experts at the Addiction Research Foundation in Toronto (Cappell *et al.*, 1986).

Griffiths and Weerts (1997) concluded in another review that the reinforcing effect of benzodiazepines was increased in subjects with a history of previous self-administration of sedatives. Research in animals and humans provides little support for the common belief that physical dependence enhances benzodiazepine reinforcement.

Earlier, Jaffe (1985) emphasized the typical behavioural patterns of addicts. He held that addiction is 'a behavioural pattern of drug use, characterized by overwhelming involvement with the use of a drug (compulsive use), the securing of its supply, and a high tendency to relapse after withdrawal'. Bejerot (1972) went even further in describing addiction as an artificially induced drive on a par with aggression and sexuality.

With regard to prescribed medications, such addictive behaviour was nearly always found in polydrug addicts who misused benzodiazepines as part of a career based primarily on stimulants, opioids or alcohol. Street addicts chose benzodiazepines to attenuate the withdrawal symptoms of stimulant abuse, and to potentiate the effects of opioids when barbiturates were not available (Allgulander, 1996).

Clinical studies at the Addiction Research Foundation in Toronto contrasted some of these patient risk factors. Patients were studied with DSM-IV benzodiazepine dependence and were admitted owing to substantial impairment. Of 30 such admissions, 25 were found to be polydrug abusers, 13 had an antisocial personality disorder, eight an avoidant personality disorder and five a borderline personality disorder (Busto *et al.*, 1996a). Another patient population was also studied (Romach *et al.*, 1995): 34 non-dependent patients who sought assistance because they wished to discontinue after having been treated with benzodiazepines for at least 3 months. Most had used low or moderate doses, and had gone from regular to use as required.

Physical dependence

Physical dependence is often confused with addiction (Lader and File, 1987). The two concepts were discussed by the DSM-IIIR committee on benzodiazepine dependence (1987):

'It should be noted that there are people who continue to take benzodiazepine medication according to a physician's direction for a legitimate medical indication such as symptoms of chronic severe anxiety. These people would not ordinarily develop symptoms that meet with the criteria for dependence, because they are not preoccupied with obtaining the substance, and its use does not interfere with their performing their normal social or occupational roles. On the contrary, the benzodiazepines may make normal functioning possible. Nevertheless, these people are likely to develop 'physical dependence' on benzodiazepines, in the pharmacological sense, because a withdrawal syndrome would ensue if the use of the substance were terminated abruptly.'

The diverging opinions regarding benzodiazepine toxicity led the American Psychiatric Association (1990) to appoint a task force. It reported on, among other things, benzodiazepine withdrawal symptoms. Based on the available studies, the task force defined a discontinuance syndrome with three components: rebound, recurrence, and withdrawal. Nocebo (negative expectations), one might add, may aggravate this syndrome.

Symptoms that were experienced in the wake of long-term anxiolytic benzodiazepine treatment were photophobia, perceptual hyperacusis, auditory and visual hypersensitivity, tinnitus, tremor, myoclonus, seizures, confusion, delusions and hallucinations. Following termination of maintenance treatment with hypnotic benzodiazepines, there were reports of increased sleep latency, REM sleep rebound, rebound insomnia, and daytime rebound anxiety. One study found that 15–25% of those treated regularly for more than 12 months developed a withdrawal syndrome, although only a small percentage reported major distress (Busto *et al.*, 1986).

To what extent these symptoms occurred prior to benzodiazepine treatment is unknown. Nearly all studies were done in retrospect. Neither are symptoms of this nature specific to this class of medications. Discontinuance syndromes are also recognized for neuroleptics, tricyclics, corticosteroids, beta-receptor stimulants and blockers, and most recently the serotonin-specific reuptake inhibitors (SSRIs) and venlafaxine (Zitman, 1999).

A test of subject and item validity of the DSM-IIIR (*Diagnostic and Statistical Manual of Mental Disorders*) and ICD-10 (International Classification of Diseases, 10th revision; WHO, 1992) dependence criteria was made on 599 benzodiazepine users by means of Rasch modelling (Kan *et al.*, 1998). Only subsets of the criteria met the homogeneity requirement, calling for a redefining of the constructs. Unrealistic rates (40–97%) of dependence were found among benzodiazepine-treated patients (Kan *et al.*, 1997).

Tolerance

In typical patients, dose escalation is rare. On the contrary, it is often necessary to encourage patients to take sufficiently high doses to be efficacious (Romach *et al.*, 1992). Tolerance develops to the anticonvulsant and sedative effects, and to a lesser degree, if at all, to the hypnotic and anxiolytic effects (Hutchinson *et al.*, 1996).

Certain individuals may be prone to develop tolerance, as measured with saccadic eye movements, which is a clue to identifying patients who react idiosyncratically to treatment (Glue *et al.*, 1993). Daughters of alcoholics responded with a pleasant mood when given alprazolam in an experimental study (Ciraulo *et al.*, 1996). This approach to identify aberrant responders is supported by the current view of addiction as a brain disorder (Leshner, 1997).

POINTS OF CONTROVERSY

Effects of regulatory intervention

The exposure to benzodiazepines varies widely within Europe. The cultural acceptance of medicating for common colds, insomnia, pain or anxiety is much higher in France and Belgium for example than in Finland or Sweden. Regulatory attitudes also differ, although they may become more harmonized within the European Union. Sweden scheduled the benzodiazepines as narcotics in 1971, while the World Health Organization did so only in 1984. Numbered prescriptions, similar to bank cheques, are mandatory in Sweden for benzodiazepines to enable pharmacists to monitor both physicians and patients and to report deviant prescribing patterns to a disciplinary inquiry. It is therefore not surprising that in Sweden utilization of benzodiazepines is lowest in the world.

There was a 57% reduction in benzodiazepine prescribing in New York state after regulation in 1989 that provided a copy of each prescription to the federal Drug Enforcement Agency (Reidenberg, 1991). In parallel, meprobamate prescriptions rose 130%, hydroxyzine 16%, chloral hydrate 127% and buspirone 124%. The street price for 1 mg alprazolam rose from $1.50 to $8.50, and 10 mg diazepam from $2 to $6. A more extensive analysis, including intensive care for overdosing with more toxic compounds, concluded that the net effect of the regulation was more likely to jeopardize than to safeguard public health (Woods *et al.*, 1992). A government task force could reach a consensus on the utility of such drugs diversion control systems because most studies were weak in design (National Institute on Drug Abuse, 1993).

What if benzodiazepines are made available without prescription? A study in Santiago, Chile, tried to assess the preventive effect of prescribing versus over-the-counter purchase in pharmacies (Busto *et al.*, 1996b). A survey was made among 1500 residents where benzodiazepines can be purchased without a prescription. Some 6% reported daily treatment with benzodiazepines for at least 12 months. The rate of DSM-IIIR benzodiazepine dependence was not affected by whether the medication was obtained by prescription or over the counter.

The concept of *rebound insomnia* was launched by one sleep researcher in 1988, and it gained attention in professional gatherings and in the media.

A critical review found this work to be 'based on poor methodology, inadequate test measures, improper interpretation of data, and the multiple publication of the same results' (Jonas, 1992).

Triazolam, synthesized by the Upjohn Company in 1969, was removed from the market by the British regulatory authority in 1991, and subsequently by the Norwegian and Finnish authorities. This was because of concerns over peculiar neuropsychiatric reactions thought to be specifically caused by triazolam. The European Community appointed a task force which quickly recommended a review of all short-acting hypnotics. The bulk of the evidence indicated that high doses of any short-acting hypnotic had the propensity to induce anterograde amnesia and paradoxical mental reactions in high-risk individuals with personality disorders. The media coverage was extensive, and the world's most common hypnotic medication was again 'on trial' (Lasagna, 1980). Triazolam quickly fell into disrepute and patients were switched to zolpidem and zopiclone. The lynching of triazolam by the British regulatory authorities triggered an ethics statement by the European Sleep Research Society (Borbely et al., 1991):
'We are of the opinion that much of the criticism (against benzodiazepine hypnotics) has been poorly informed and while we adhere to the view that drugs should never be unnecessarily prescribed ... doctors have an obligation to help and comfort their patients and not discipline them.'

Personal comment

I could not agree more. It is saddening that patients with morbid anxiety and insomnia amenable to benzodiazepine treatment have been stigmatized as being dependent, and made to suffer unnecessarily in the overzealous interest of prevention. Much of the effort spent on reducing benzodiazepine treatments could better have been invested in neurobiological research on the molecular aspects of addiction.

Benzodiazepines can be part of a polydrug-abusing career characterized by compulsive drug-seeking behaviour. The natural history of such addictive behaviour is dismal. It is literally of vital importance that addicted patients are taken care of by specialists. When addiction also involves prescribed medications, one may expect even more psychopathology than in primary alcohol or street drug addiction, and even higher degrees of self-destructive behaviour. It is not sufficient in such patients to withhold psychoactive medications in the belief that these are the culprits. Just as important is to conduct proper psychiatric diagnosing and institute adjunctive or alternative measures. When we fail to alter addictive behaviour, again it is wrong to conclude that the medication is at fault.

REFERENCES

Allgulander, C. (1986). History and current status of sedative-hypnotic drug use and abuse. *Acta Psychiatr Scand* **73**, 465–478.

Allgulander, C. (1996). Addiction on prescribed sedative-hypnotics. *Hum Psychopharmacol* **11**, S49–S54.

Allgulander, C., Ljungberg, L. and Fisher, L.D. (1987). Long-term prognosis in addiction on sedative and hypnotic drugs analyzed with the Cox regression model. *Acta Psychiatr Scand* **75**, 521–531.

American Psychiatric Association (1990). *Benzodiazepine Dependence, Toxicity, and Abuse*. A Task Force Report. American Psychiatric Association,Washington, DC.

Bejerot, N. (1972). *Addiction. An Artificially Induced Drive*. Charles C. Thomas Publisher, Springfield, IL, pp. 1–77.

Bell, C. and Nutt, D.J. (1995). Benzodiazepines in the treatment of anxiety. In: Nutt, D.J. and Mendelson, W.B. (Eds), *Hypnotics and Anxiolytics*. Baillière Tindall, London, pp. 391–411.

Borbely, A.A., Åkerstedt, T., Benoit, O. *et al.* (1991). Hypnotics and sleep physiology: a consensus report. *Eur Arch Psychiatr Clin Neurosci* **241**, 13–21.

Busto, U.E., Sellers, E.M., Naranjo, C.A., Cappell, H.D., Sanchez, C.M. and Simpkins, J. (1986). Patterns of benzodiazepine abuse and dependence. *Br J Addict* **81**, 87–94.

Busto, U.E., Romach, M.K. and Sellers, E.M. (1996a). Multiple drug use and psychiatric comorbidity in patients admitted to the hospital with severe benzodiazepine dependence. *J Clin Psychopharmacol* **16**, 51–57.

Busto, U.E., Ruiz, I., Busto, M. and Gacitua, A. (1996b). Benzodiazepine use in Chile: impact of availability on use, abuse, and dependence. *J Clin Psychopharmacol* **16**, 363–372.

Cappell, H.D., Sellers, E.M. and Busto, U. (1986). Benzodiazepines as drugs of abuse and dependence. In: Cappell, H.D., Glaser, F., Israel, Y. *et al.* (Eds), *Research Advances in Alcohol and Drug Problems, Vol. 9*. Plenum Press, New York, pp. 53–126.

Ciraulo, D.A., Sarid, S.O., Knapp, C., Ciraulo, A.M., Greenblatt, D.J. and Shader, R.I. (1996). Liability to alprazolam abuse in daughters of alcoholics. *Am Psychiatry* **153**, 956–958.

Frank, J., Mattila-Evenden, M., Rydberg, U., Åsberg, M. and Bergman, U. (1996). DSM IV profile of benzodiazepine users claiming compensation. Poster, International Symposium on Pharmacoepidemiology, Budapest, 1996.

Glue, P., Wilson, S.J. and Nutt, D. (1993). The role of the benzodiazepine receptor in anxiety. In: Hallström, C. (Ed.), *Benzodiazepine Dependence*. Oxford University Press, Oxford, pp. 71–94.

Griffiths, R.R. and Weerts, E.M. (1997). Benzodiazepine self-administration in humans and laboratory animals – implications for problems of long-term use and abuse. *Psychopharmacology* **134**, 1–37.

Hollister, L.E., Müller-Oerlinghausen, B., Rickels, M. and Shader, R.I. (1993). Clinical uses of benzodiazepines. *J Clin Psychopharmacol* **13** (suppl 1), 1S–169S.

Hutchinson, M.A., Smith, P.F. and Darlington, C.L. (1996). The behavioural and neuronal effects of the chronic administration of benzodiazepine anxiolytic and hypnotic drugs. *Prog Neurobiol* **49**, 73–97.

Ideström, C.-M. (1969). Behandling av oro, ångest och sömnsvårigheter. 4. Missbruk och olycksfall. *Läkartidningen* **66** (suppl 1), 73–76.

Jaffe, J.H. (1985). Drug addiction and drug abuse. In: Gilman, A.G., Goodman, L.S. and Gilman, A. (Eds), *The Pharmacological Basis of Therapeutics*, pp. 535–584.

Jonas, J.M. (1992). Idiosyncratic side effects of short half-life benzodiazepine hypnotic: fact or fancy? *Hum Psychopharmacol* **7**, 205–216.

Kan, C.C., Breteler, M.H. and Zitman, F.G. (1997). High prevalence of benzodiazepine dependence in out-patient users, based on the DSM-III-R and ICD-10 criteria. *Acta Psychiatr Scand* **96**, 85–93.

Kan, C.C., Breteler, M.H., van der Ven, A. and Zitman, F.G. (1998). An evaluation of DSM-III-R and ICD-10 benzodiazepine dependence criteria using Rasch modelling. *Addiction* **93**, 349–359.

Kräupl Taylor, F.K. (1989). The damnation of benzodiazepines. *Br J Psychiatr* **154**, 697–704.

Lader, M. (1978). Benzodiazepines – the opium of the masses? *Neuroscience* **3**, 159–165.

Lader, M. and File, S.E. (1987). The biological basis of benzodiazepine dependence. *Psychol Med* **17**, 539–547.

Lasagna, L. (1980). The Halcion story: trial by media. *Lancet* **ii**, 815–816.

Le Guillant, L. (1930). La toxicomanie barbiturique. Thèse, Paris.

Leshner, A.I. (1997). Addiction is a brain disease and it matters. *Science* **278**, 45–47.

Ljungberg, L. (1957). Hysteria. A clinical, prognostic and genetic study. *Acta Psychiatr Scand Suppl* **112**, 1–162.

National Institute on Drug Abuse (1993). *Impact of Prescription Drug Diversion Control Systems on Medical Practice and Patient Care.* NIDA Research Monograph 131. NIDA, Washington DC, pp. 343.

Nimb, M. (1975). Misbrug af euforiserende stoffer i Danmark i 1950' erne med efterundersögelse i 1972. Dissertation 2547, University of Copenhagen.

Pohlisch, K. and Panse, F. (1934). *Schlutmittelmissbrauch.* Thieme, Leipzig.

Reidenberg, M.M. (1991). Effect of the requirement for triplicate prescriptions for benzodiazepines in New York State. *Clin Pharmacol Therapeut* **50**, 129–131.

Retterstöl, N. and Sund, A. (1964). Drug addiction and habituation. An investigation with personal follow-up of 122 drug-addicted and habituated patients previously treated in a psychiatric clinical department. *Acta Psychiatr Scand Suppl* **179**, 1–120.

Romach, M.K., Somer, G.R., Sobell, M.B., Kaplan, H.L. and Sellers, E.M. (1992). Characteristics of long-term alprazolam users in the community. *J Clin Psychopharmacol* **12**, 316–321.

Romach, M., Busto, U., Somer, G., Kaplan, H.L. and Sellers, E. (1995). Clinical aspects of chronic use of alprazolam and lorazepam. *Am J Psychiatr* **152**, 1161–1167.

Royal College of Psychiatrists (1997). *Benzodiazepines: Risks, Benefits or Dependence. A Re-evaluation.* Council Report CR59. Royal College of Psychiatrists, London, pp. 1–9.

Swanson, D.W.R., Weddige, R.L. and Morse, R.M. (1973). Abuse of prescription drugs.*Mayo Clin Proc* **48**, 359–367.

Szasz, T. (1974). *Ceremonial Chemistry.* Anchor Press/Doubleday, New York, p. 15.

Vanggaard, T. (1988). Angsttilstande og deres behandling. *Nord Psykiatr Tidsskrift* **40**, 421–424.

Whitlock, F.A. (1970). The syndrome of barbiturate dependence. *Med J Aust*, 391–404.

Wissler, W. (1969). Pathogenese und Prognose der Hypnotica-abhängigkeit. *Schweiz Arch Neurol Neurochir Psychiatr* **104**, 389–425.

Woods, J.H., Katz, J.L. and Winger, G. (1987). Abuse liability of benzodiazepines, *Pharmacol Rev* **39**, 251–419.

Woods, J.H., Katz, J.L. and Winger, G. (1992). Benzodiazepines: use, abuse and consequences. *Pharmacol Rev* **44**, 151–347.

World Health Organization (1996). *Rational Use of Benzodiazepines.* WHO, Geneva.

Zitman, F.G. (1999). Strategies for the discontinuation of psychotropic drugs: at last but not at least. *Curr Med Lit Psychiatr* **10**, 1–7.

Index

Neuronal damage, in status epilepticus 75, 81
Neuron-specific enolase, serum, in status
    epilepticus 81
Neurosteroids, *see* Steroids
New England Journal of Medicine 50–52
Nicotine 35
Nitrazepam
    in childhood epilepsy 50, 88, 89
    dose equivalence 50
    in epilepsy 66
    hypnotic use 38
    for infantile spasms 89, 90, 92
    in Lennox–Gastaut syndrome 93
    prescribing patterns 44, 149

Obsessional states 46
Opioid abuse 151
Opium 37, 42–43, 147–148
Over-the-counter purchasing 153
Oxazepam 50, 149

Paediatric epilepsy, *see* Childhood epilepsy
Panic disorder 42, 51, 52
Paraldehyde 43
Parasomnias 30, 31, 32, 34
Paroxysmal dystonic choreoathetosis (PDC)
    127, 128
Paroxysmal exercise-induced dyskinesia
    (PED) 127, 128
Paroxysmal kinesigenic choreoathetosis
    (PKC) 127–128
Paroxysmal nocturnal (hypnogenic)
    dyskinesia 127
Partial agonists 5–6
    abercarnil as 11
    as anxiolytics 5–6, 9
    mechanisms of action 7, 8
    see also Clobazam
Partial inverse agonists 7
Partial seizures, drug-resistant 93
Passengers, airplane 55
    intercontinental travel 55–58
    managing sleep disturbance 60–61
    use of hypnotics 62–64
Pentobarbitone, in status epilepticus 82
Perceptual representation system (PRS) 21
Performance, time zone changes and 60
Personality disorders 46, 148, 151
Phaclofen 3
Pharmacoeconomics 131–146
Pharmacokinetics, acute administration 77–78
Pharmacological properties 1–16
Phenobarbitone
    clobazam interactions 91
    in myoclonic disorders 125
    in status epilepticus 82, 94
Phenothiazines 47
Phenytoin
    in childhood epilepsy 90–91, 107

clobazam interaction 119
    in movement disorders 128
    in status epilepticus 79, 82
Phobic disorders 42, 46
Pilocarpine-induced status epilepticus 76
Piracetam, in myoclonic disorders 125
Polymorphous epilepsy, severe 93
Polypharmacy, rational 70
Polysomnography, for aircrew 62
Polytherapy, in epilepsy 70–71, 131
Post-anoxic myoclonus 66, 122
Potassium bromide 43
Premedication 17
Prescribing, benzodiazepine
    Committee on Safety of Medicine
        guidelines 45–46
    contemporary review 48–50
    impact of guidelines 46–48
    patterns 44–45, 51, 149
    regulatory interventions 153–154
Primary care
    benzodiazepine prescribing 46
    sleep disorders in 29–40
Primidone, in myoclonic disorders 125
Priming 21
    conceptual 21
    perceptual 21
Prisoners 47–48
Progabide 2
Propofol, in status epilepticus 82
Pseudo-dementia, drug-induced 24–25
Psychiatric disorders
    sleep disturbance 30, 31, 32
    see also Anxiety; Depression; Psychosis
Psychoactive drugs
    misuse, *see* Misuse, drug
    prescribing practice 47
Psychosis 147
    clobazam-induced 68–69
    post-ictal 71
Pyrazolopyridines 5

Quality of life (QOL)
    assessment in epilepsy 131–133
    in cost-effectiveness study 135–136, 141
Quality of Life Assessment by Construct
    Analysis (QoLASCA) 132, 135
Quality of Life Assessment Schedule
    (QOLAS) 135–136
    in cost-effectiveness study 139–140, 141

Receptor-reserve hypothesis 12
Rectal diazepam, *see* Diazepam, rectal
Regulatory interventions 153–154
Reinforcement 150–151
Repertory Grid Technique (RGT) 132, 135
Restless legs syndrome 62
Reticular formation, in startle syndromes 126
RO 15-4513 7, 8